HAVING SURGERY?

Using Music to Reduce Anxiety and Pain Perception

A GUIDE FOR PATIENTS AND HEALTH CARE PROVIDERS

Alice Hudnall Cash PhD, LCSW

Trademark notices / Patent notices:

The Surgical Serenity Solution's proprietary patented process is founded on the idea that music affects the body profoundly, even when the patient is asleep, because of well documented phenomenon known as rhythmic entrainment.

U. S. Patent #7,431,689 B2 (October 7, 2008)

Printed version ISBN: 978-1-7342823-0-6

First Printing: 2020

Surgical Serenity Solutions

2822 Frankfort Avenue

Louisville KY 40206

P: 502.419.1698

F. 502.895.7688

DrAlice@SurgicalSerenitySolutions.com

Ordering Information:

For information about special discounts available for bulk purchases, sales promotions, fund-raising and educational needs, contact Surgical Serenity Solutions at 1-502.419.1698 or email DrAlice@SurgicalSerenitySolutions.com.

Visit: www.surgicalserenitysolutions.com/

Praise from Users of Surgical Serenity Solutions Music Apps

"The surgical headphones were great, and the nurses were very receptive to the idea; the music was very helpful during surgical prep and throughout the surgery. The doctors were enthusiastic too! I'm already home and the surgery went well. The surgical headphones were a big hit and I will definitely recommend them to my friends and family."

- Kathy Baucom, Louisville KY

"My knee surgery was not nearly as bad as I feared because the beautiful music on your headphones calmed me down immediately and made me feel as though I was somewhere else, where everything was OK!"

- Elizabeth Clifford, Louisville KY

"Before my abdominal aortic aneurysm surgery, I was told that surgery would take 4-5 hours; it took less than 2! I was also told that I'd be in ICU for 3-4 days and I was out after one night! The music was beautiful and calming."

- Jim Wilhelm, Louisville KY

"Dr. Cash, thank you so much for helping me choose the perfect music for my hip replacement surgery. The procedure went exceptionally smoothly and knowing that I had music that I loved made everything easier. I plan to be back on my cross-country skis in February."

- Barb E., patient

"My son's surgery was yesterday. He wore the headset for two hours before surgery and during the procedure. Unlike his last surgery, all went well. Lots of people were involved to make sure he reacted well to the anesthesia and other medicines provided. They were very happy to let him use the headphones in the operating room. He went into surgery thinking the headset would be helpful in keeping him calm and needing less anesthesia, and he did remain calm after coming around post-op. We believe your music was integral to his good experience. Many thanks! "

- Faith Nuygen, mother of patient

Free Checklist of Reasons to Use Music to Reduce Anxiety and Pain Perception During Surgery and Recovery

Are you thinking of using music to reduce anxiety and pain perception for an upcoming medical procedure? You may need to convince your doctor.

Download this free checklist of information that you can give your doctor. It will help immensely!

Visit: www.surgicalserenitysolutions.com/free-checklist

The Surgical Serenity Solutions App is now available for iPhone, iTouch, and Android devices. The following playlists are featured:

- Classical Blend

- Jazz

- New Age

- Lullabies

- Memory Care

Users can select one or multiple playlists. Playlists are designed for continuous play throughout the procedure, regardless of length.

We recommend that patients listen to playlists using earbuds or headphones so that extraneous noise and conversations are eliminated.

Visit the Surgical Serenity Solutions website for direct links to purchase the app of your choice. Click here or type this URL into your device browser:

www.surgicalserenitysolutions.com/digital-products/

DISCLAIMER

This book is not intended as a substitute for the medical advice of physicians or other healthcare professionals.

Although the author has made every effort to ensure that the information in this book was correct at press time, the author does not assume and hereby disclaims any liability to any party for any loss, damage, or disruption caused by errors or omissions, whether such errors or omissions result from negligence, accident, or any other cause.

Surgical Serenity Solutions is not liable for any information provided with regards to recommendations and usage of music to aid health-related issues.

The products and claims made about specific products on or through this site have not been evaluated by the United States Food and Drug Administration and are not approved to diagnose, treat, cure, or prevent disease.

This book, and linked websites, are not intended to provide diagnosis, treatment, or medical advice. Products, services, information and other content provided including information that may be provided directly or by linking to third-party websites are provided for informational purposes only.

Some names and identifying details have been changed to protect the privacy of individuals.

DEDICATION

To my mentor and guide in all things Music Medicine, Dr. Arthur Harvey (1938-2017.) Arthur has been my unflagging encourager and supporter since 1990, when I went to hear him speak at the University of Louisville School of Medicine. He was a beloved college music professor at both Eastern Kentucky University and the University of Hawaii, Manoa. Dr. Harvey was also a dedicated church musician and performer on dozens of musical instruments as well as having a beautiful voice. He left us too soon, but his kindness to me and his encouragement to "go deep" in the pursuit to bring music into surgery will never be forgotten.

Also, to my many friends in the field of Music Therapy, who have listened to my ideas and stories and been consistently and unflaggingly positive and encouraging! Dr. Barbara Wheeler, MT-BC; Lisa Gallagher, MT-BC; Ellen Cool, MT-BC.

TABLE OF CONTENTS

FOREWORD

Many of us may know, whether it's on an intuitive or cognitive level, that listening to music can help us relax. Many may also know that listening to music can provide powerful relief from pain. Others also know that music can actually assist the healing process.

However, our ability to listen to music during situations when it might truly be needed, such as in the operating room, has often been limited by the equipment that existed. Until the advent of personal stereo system, which began with the cassette playing Sony Walkman and other similar devices around 1980, it was not possible to listen to music without disturbing others. Since then, the world of the personal stereo has rapidly blossomed, moving from cassette to CD players, then mp3s players and the like. It now seems possible to literally have a majority of the world's music available on a device that might be only a few inches in size.

On a physiological (and emotional) level, certain types of music can lower our heart rate and respiration, help reduce stress, release endorphins and reduce pain. Therapeutic music can do so much more—which Alice Cash so wonderfully details in this book, *Having Surgery? Using Music to Reduce Anxiety and Pain Perception*. In addition, music can lower the need for anesthesia. Most important is finding the proper music to use that will work for each person. Of equal importance, finding the proper device that will unobtrusively offer playback and function properly during the listener's surgical experience is vital.

Some years ago, I was undergoing a minor surgical procedure which required anesthesia. I had much knowledge of how music could help induce relaxation and healing and created a CD of music that I knew would benefit my experience. I brought along a portable CD player, turned it on and as the anesthetic began to take effect, I eased into a truly deep state of bliss. This lasted for about a minute before one of the people in the operating room accidentally hit the CD player and disconnected my headphones. I won't describe my awareness of the music stopping, but it was not pleasant. In addition, I hadn't received enough aesthetic to make me fully unconscious and I was still able to hear the activities going on in the OR with the doctor and staff. It made a lasting impression on me. I understood that the need to have some sort of music playback system that wasn't intrusive and could be utilized during the surgical procedure was imperative. Since that time, I've known of others who have had similar experiences or worse. Some have even discovered that their expensive equipment had mysteriously disappeared during the procedure.

When Dr. Alice Cash presented the concept of her *Surgical Serenity Solutions Headphones* to me, I immediately understood their brilliance. Here was a playback system that actually consisted totally and solely of headphones which could be played without impedance during a surgical procedure. There were no cords, wires or separate player that could interfere with a medical procedure. And which (better yet!) offered a variety of soothing types of music to please even the most discriminant musical listener.

Alice Cash's *Surgical Serenity Solutions Headphones* are truly a gift for all. Her book, "Having Surgery? Using Music to Reduce Anxiety and Pain Perception," is a well-documented exploration of how and why music can be effective during surgery and recovery. It addresses some of the challenges that patients may encounter when trying to bring music playback systems into the operating room. This excellent book explains includes how to introduce the subject of listening to music and its profound benefits during surgery to the medical community. Many doctors and other hospital staff members simply don't know about the extraordinary ability of music to relax, reduce pain, and to assist the healing process. I trust this book will help and be of great service. I trust that more and more people will be entering the operating room while being privately bathed in the sonorous and soothing vibrations coming from the *Surgical Serenity Solution Headphones*. How extraordinary that would be!

Jonathan Goldman
7 Secrets of Sound Healing, author
Grammy-Nominated Composer in New Age Category

When Dr. Cash asked me to write the forward to this book, I was thrilled to accept! Of course, I am honored to be asked, but more than that, I am thrilled for you, the reader. In this book, you are going to discover how music can be a strategic tool in preparing for surgery. You will learn about the profound power of rhythmic entrainment, which has been a tool of music therapists for years, but was never applied to music for the surgical patient. She will show you, page by page, how rhythmic entrainment, as used in her unique playlists, can reduce your anxiety and pain perception. Because you see, Dr. Cash has distilled the essence of research in nursing, anesthesia, surgery, and music therapy to using specific music in a particular way that will allow you to achieve these results and more.

If you are facing a surgical procedure or if you simply want a proven method to reduce anxiety and pain perception, then this book is for you. If you are a healthcare professional, this book can assist you in using a scientifically verified method that will help your patients reduce their perioperative, operative and post-operative anxiety and pain, while lowering the need for potentially addictive pain medications. And if you are a hospital or clinic administrator, the use of Surgical Serenity Solution's patented system can lower costs while improving patient satisfaction.

As a former healthcare provider, myself (I worked as a PA in Emergency and Occupational Medicine for over two decades) I can attest to the often debilitating anxiety many patients go through when they face a surgical procedure. This puts a huge strain on patients and their families, and can many times lead to unwanted complications from the procedure.

As a talented and respected musician, seasoned psychotherapist and educator, Dr. Alice Cash has devoted her life and her work to the relief of this suffering. This book is the culmination of those years of devotion. The information and methods she lays out in this book will provide you with specific ways to use music to manage your or your patients anxiety and pain when approaching surgical or medical procedures.

Ellen Britt, Physician Assistant, Ed.D

READ ME FIRST

Do you experience fear and anxiety before, during, and after surgical procedures? If yes, know that you are not alone. Making matters worse, many patients also worry about related issues, including:

- Adverse reactions to anesthesia

- The probability of increased pain and lengthy recovery time

- Risk of addiction to post-operative pain-relieving drugs, especially opioids

The drug-free solution offered by Surgical Serenity Solutions explained in this book was developed specifically with people like you in mind. In these pages, you'll discover a simple, natural system you can use to reduce pain perception and side-effects of surgery…plus recover in less time.

Before we jump in, a simple explanation of what the term *"rhythmic entrainment"* means is in order. Rhythmic entrainment is key to why and how the music delivery system developed by Surgical Serenity Solutions works. This system is available to you today using our headphones or downloading one of our patented specially created music tracks to your mobile phone.

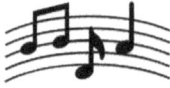

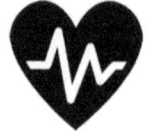

Rhythmic entrainment is a well-documented phenomenon in which a person's breathing and heart rate synchronizes to an external rhythm, such as music, a clock ticking, or a drumbeat.

I am Dr. Alice Cash, founder of Surgical Serenity Solutions. In addition to being one of the world's few clinical musicologists, I've brought over 40 years of experience as a college professor, clinical therapist, international speaker, researcher, solo and chamber music performer and composer into my work and product development.

Music is my passion. Using music to help ease the pain and suffering of others is my mission.

INTRODUCTION

The use of music to alleviate human pain and suffering is as ancient as a mother singing to her newborn. For over two thousand years, people around the world have been aware of music's soothing abilities. However, understanding just how music affects the mind and physical human body was a mystery.

Extensive modern research has made great strides in our understanding of how music affects the mind-body connection. Researchers now know how specific music tempi work to calm the rapidly beating heart and shallow breathing.

In medical language, music is known as a natural anxiolytic agent. Anxiolytic means "anxiety relieving." Anti-anxiety medications are artificial anxiolytic agents. Just as a driver needn't know all the mechanics of an engine before starting a car, shifting into gear, and rolling down the highway, it's not essential that you understand all the science behind how music, especially specific styles and tempos of music, work to "entrain" the breathing and rapid heartbeat that are present with fear and anxiety.

Recall from the *Read Me First* section that "**rhythmic entrainment**" is a well-documented phenomenon in which a person's breathing and heart rate synchronize to an external rhythm, such as music, a clock ticking, or a drumbeat.

Surgical Serenity Solutions playlists are specially designed to facilitate this synchronization by using the most effective tempo, melodies, and genres.

What is worth understanding are the many benefits this drug-free solution provides patients struggling with fear and anxiety when facing medical procedures, especially surgery with a lengthy, painful recovery.

Some of the benefits reported by patients using Surgical Serenity Solutions' headphones and proprietary music are:

- *Calming effects pre- and post-procedure*

- *Greatly reduced anxiety level*

- *Reduced amount of anesthesia*

- *Reduced side effects from anesthesia*

- *Reduced time to discharge and recovery time*

- *Reduced need for post-procedure opioids*

- *Improved patient experience/satisfaction*

Who Can Benefit from Rhythmic Entrainment?

> Patients

Whether facing a dental procedure, major or minor surgery, or a cosmetic procedure at a medical spa, rhythmic entrainment is a proven method to help patients relax, minimize the perception of pain, and even reduce the need for painkillers following the procedure.

> Parents and Caregivers

Whether in their infancy or golden years, people of all ages can benefit from rhythmic entrainment in their day-to-day lives. Surgical Serenity Solution's proprietary lullabies can help prepare children for bedtime, while our memory care playlist can help soothe seniors with the familiar sounds of their youth.

> Hospitals, Surgery Centers, Dental Offices and Med Spas

When it comes to differentiating medical services from the competition, an enhanced patient experience goes hand in hand with positive outcomes. The Surgical Serenity Solution headphone system and patented playlists help provide medical facilities with an affordable way to demonstrate your commitment to patient comfort and care.

> Physicians and Clinicians

As a physician or member of the patient care team, you want the best possible outcomes for your patients. Providing a personalized experience using Surgical Serenity Solutions playlists has helped improved patient satisfaction and reduce recovery times.

At the time publication, patients have used Surgical Serenity Solutions' patented music in a wide variety of clinical procedures, including:

- Abdominal aortic aneurysm
- Breast biopsy
- Cardiac catheterization lab procedures (e.g. pacemaker implantation)
- Cardiac surgery (e.g. aortic aneurysm bypass, open heart procedures)
- Caesarian Section
- Chemotherapy
- Colonoscopy
- Dental surgery

- Eye Surgery (e.g., cataract, glaucoma, LASIK, macular degeneration)

- General anxiety (e.g., routine shots, exams)

- Hysterectomy

- Joint replacement (e.g., ankle, hip, knee, shoulder)

- Labor and Delivery

- Lithotripsy

- Mastectomy

- Pediatric heart surgery

Guide to Using This Book

This book is divided into three main sections:

- **Part I: A Patient's Guide to Using Music to Reduce Fear and Anxiety During Surgery and Recovery,** is devoted to providing patients and caregivers basic information on how listening to specific types of music can help reduce fear, pain, and anxiety before, during, and after surgery and other medical procedures.

- **Part II: Insights into the History and Science of Using Music During Medical Procedures,** dives deeper into the history and science of using music for health care benefits. Some readers will appreciate this fascinating information. Other readers will be happy to skip this section altogether and focus exclusively on Part I and the advantages of using a pair of Surgical Serenity Solutions' headphones and proprietary music playlists for personal and family use.

- **Part III: How Hospitals, Clinics, and Medical Professionals are using Surgical Serenity Solutions** provides specific information, research and development, and case studies of special interest to hospitals, doctors, dental offices. clinics, and medical professionals. Dr. Alice Cash, founder and CEO of Surgical Serenity Solutions, has worked extensively with interested facilities, doctors, and researchers on numerous field studies.

Surgical Serenity Solutions was founded by Dr. Alice Cash, a clinical musicologist, therapist, and accomplished concert pianist. A clinical researcher at the University of Louisville School of Medicine during the '90's, her clinical work at the University of Louisville led to her career in Music Medicine.

In 2008, she received a US patent on her unique process for using music in the perioperative period. Today, her solutions are used by leading hospitals, plastic surgery practices and patients in the US and around the world.

Surgical Serenity Solutions continues to collaborate with a team of technical and healthcare advisors including physicians, psychologists, music therapists and business advisors across the U.S., in Europe and in the Middle East.

See our website to learn more about our headphones and how to download our patented music playlists. Here's the link:
www.surgicalserenitysolutions.com/products

ABOUT THE AUTHOR

Dr. Alice Cash is one of the world's few clinical musicologists. She brings to her work over 40 years of experience as a college professor, clinical musicologist, clinical social worker, international speaker, writer, and solo and chamber music performer and composer.

Based in Louisville, Kentucky, Dr. Cash began her work in Music Medicine in 1990 at the University of Louisville School of Medicine under the guidance of Dr Arthur Harvey, a music medicine practitioner, Dr. Leah Dickstein, a psychiatrist and Dr. Joel Elkes, an internationally known psychiatrist. She travels the globe speaking to doctors and patients alike, teaching them about the benefits of music with surgery.

In 2008, she received a U.S. Patent on her unique system for adding music to the surgical procedure, using preloaded headphones with proprietary music, chosen to engage rhythmic entrainment in the patient and reduce anxiety, pain, and medication requirements, resulting in a faster recovery and a safer procedure. Her special music playlists are now available in app form for download to smart phones.

Additional information about Dr. Cash, along with access to her complete curriculum vitae (CV) please visit her website or see the *More About Dr. Alice Cash* section of this book.

"Dr. Alice H. has as many facets as a well-cut diamond. She is an educated and experienced professional musician as well as a well-respected professional counselor and businesswoman. I had the privilege to know Dr Alice when she first conceived of the idea to use the healing powers of music for surgery patients. My wife experienced the positive benefits of music to aid her through two complicated surgeries successfully. I recommend the power of Dr Alice's headphones and music."

- Jack Allen *SPHR, Senior Consultant and owner,*
JCA CONSULTING LLC

PREFACE

How I Became Interested in Using Music for Surgery

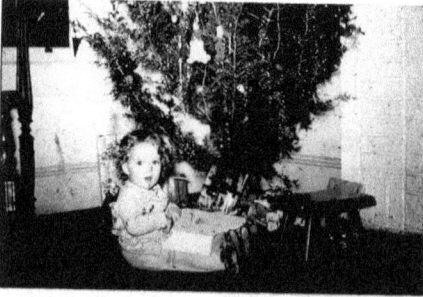

Alice's first piano recital, age 19 months

I have loved music for as long as I can remember. By the time I was 2 years old, I was singing little songs that I had learned at home and nursery school. My grandmother bought me my very own record player and a stack of records when I was 3, and I spent hours playing those records, singing and dancing to them. I started picking out tunes on the piano at age 3 but was not allowed to have piano lessons until I was 8 years old.

By age 14, I had become very serious about music and playing classical piano. I knew then that I wanted to major in music and be a professional musician, both performing and teaching. I was very fortunate to have teachers such as Edward Kilenyi at Florida State University, Lee Luvisi at University of Louisville, and Ilonka Deckers in Milan Italy. After receiving my B.M and M.M in piano performance, I married and started a family, but continued teaching and performing in local colleges, such as Southern Wesleyan College, the University of Georgia, the University of Louisville, and Indiana University Southeast.

In 1990, I earned my PhD in musicology and was immediately offered a new position at the School of Medicine, University of Louisville. My job was to conduct clinical research on the healing power of music with different populations. It was here where I was introduced to the concept of using music with people undergoing surgery of all kinds. At the same time, I was studying the use of music with preemies and newborns, as well as the use of music with Alzheimer's patients.

For the next 15 years, I worked with patients having surgery, giving birth, coping with a loved one with Alzheimer's or other dementia, and people recovering from chemical dependency. All of these groups benefitted from the healing powers of music in different ways, and I loved doing this work. I had also earned a master's degree in clinical social work in 1995 and in 1997 was licensed as a therapist. Music therapy, as a discipline and a degree program, had not yet come to Kentucky (where I lived) so I did my work under the supervision of Dr. Joel Elkes, Dr. Arthur Harvey, and Dr. Leah Dickstein, in the Department of Psychiatry and Behavioral Science and the Division of Arts and Medicine.

The Evolution of Surgical Serenity Solutions

In 2002, I approached the CEO of a newly built hospital here in Louisville to ask about supporting a series of CDs that I would create just for surgery. I explained that the hospital could license the CDs, branded with its own name and logo, to other hospitals around the world. She said she was intrigued with the idea, but it never happened. I was so disappointed.

In 2005, as a member, I attended a National Speakers Association conference. I had been working with patients for about 15 years by that point. Originally, we made cassette tapes for before switching to CDs with headphones plugged into a Sony Discman.

I continued working with individual patients until 2005 when I attended the Innovation Conference and had the idea to create pre-loaded headphones that would be cordless and wireless. I set to work finding a headset that could be programmed with the perfect soothing, steady tempo music for surgery. In

October of 2008, I received a U.S. Patent for my idea and began selling a "hospital model" in 2009.

It has been an exciting and rewarding journey. In 2010, I received the first Venture Sharks Grand Prize award, which allowed me to move forward with a small staff and advisory board.

In 2014, we created our "Cloud Kit" which is intended for hospitals or clinics and consists of 10 hospital-model headphones that sit in a "kit" box with a USB hub in the bottom. This allows for the headphones to be charging simultaneously. Also, it has a pop-up dispenser in the corner for disposable earpiece covers. This way the headphones can be used between patients in a busy hospital, simply by wiping the band with a disinfectant spray and changing the disposable earpiece covers.

In 2016, we got our patient-model headphones, which are cordless and programmable, with our music tracks loaded onto a micro-SD card.

In 2018, we added four new playlists and began work on a mobile app. This app has all five of our current playlists on it, as well as full access to the website:
https://www.surgicalserenitysolutions.com/products/

The website includes dozens of articles offering helpful usage tips, research findings, case studies and, I'm proud to say, many happy patient testimonials.

Our proprietary playlists are available via our mobile app. iPhone users can download from the Apple App Store and Android users from the Google Play Store.

Currently, we have five different playlists that are intended to engage entrainment and rhythmic entrainment. In other words, the music synchronizes the listener's breathing and heart rate to the tempo of the music, thus helping the listener to relax naturally, releasing built-up tension and anxiety.

The playlists are:

- Our original classical piano music, consisting of lesser-known miniatures

- Our newly commissioned jazz playlist performed by an acclaimed jazz trio

- A New Age playlist with the synthesized sounds that allow people to drift into a state of positive relaxation, while still harnessing rhythmic entrainment

- A lullaby playlist for children or adults that includes both familiar, classic lullabies plus a few contemporary lullabies

- A 'memory-care" playlist that would be familiar to the older patient. Although it does not necessarily engage rhythmic entrainment, it could benefit the older patient who is undergoing dental work, or perhaps eye surgery or joint replacement, but doesn't require general anesthesia

All of these playlists will be streamed to your Bluetooth headphones or Bluetooth earbuds. For home use, they could be played through your phone speakers, but headphones work best for engaging rhythmic entrainment.

If you experience fear and anxiety before, during, and after surgical procedures, I hope you'll download one or more of our playlists to your mobile phone soon. Or check out our personal pre-loaded headphones available on our website.

Be sure to get our free **Checklist: Questions to Ask Your Doctor**. You'll find the list of questions along with the information to download and print the checklist at the end of Chapter 1.

Also, ask your doctor or healthcare staff if they have the Surgical Serenity Solutions headphones available at the facility for patients like you to use.

May your next surgery or medical procedure find you less stressed and on the road to recovery quicker and with less pain than ever before. I encourage you to write and share your experience with me.

Thank you for your interest in reading this book, and my patented sound approach to reduced anxiety and pain perception.

Rhythmic Entrainment Playlists and Headphones from
Surgical Serenity

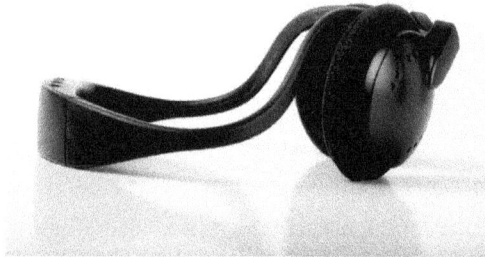

PART I

A PATIENT'S GUIDE TO USING MUSIC TO REDUCE ANXIETY AND PAIN PERCEPTION DURING SURGERY AND RECOVERY

CHAPTER 1

Sound Approach – A Better Way to Deal with Surgery

Wouldn't it be wonderful to feel relaxed and calm going into surgery rather than frazzled and fearful? And what about later as your recovery begins? Doesn't every patient hope to feel better quickly so they can move on with the more enjoyable things in life?

Whether planned or unplanned, no one wants to have surgery.

Sometimes, we don't have a choice. Perhaps you've been dreading an upcoming surgery for some time. Maybe you just found out. The unfortunate and surprise prognosis can leave you stunned, reeling from the shock. If you weren't nervous before, your anxiety level is likely on the rise causing your blood pressure to soar. It doesn't help that scheduling time for surgery and recovery will wreak havoc with your schedule, not to mention your bank account.

Many people don't like hospitals because they find them scary and overwhelming. The sterile environment, the mysterious odors and overwhelming assortment of medical tools and equipment are frightening. You feel on edge just stepping inside to visit a patient let alone checking in as one.

In this chapter, you'll learn how music can help alleviate your anxiety with the prospect of having surgery. Let's start with a review of some common fears and misconceptions about surgery. Bear with me here because it leads directly into the stories of two women who, despite dreading and anxious about their surgeries, came through them and out the other side of recovery grateful for the calming relief experienced by listening to specially created music delivered via a Surgical Serenity Solutions' headphone. One woman had unexpected surgery, the other was able to plan ahead.

Common Fears and Misconceptions About Surgery

Sometimes, when patients discover they need to have a surgical procedure, they are overcome with fear and dread fueled by questions racing through their minds. Questions such as:

- What if the surgery doesn't improve the situation?

- What if the anesthesia doesn't completely put me to sleep?

- What if I wake up before I'm supposed to?

- What if I'm allergic to the anesthesia but don't know it?

- What if I don't wake up at all?

- What if I'm feeling worse after the procedure than I was before?

Of course, all of these are real *possibilities*, but not *probabilities*. Surgery has become safer and safer as time has gone by and medicine has advanced tremendously. The fields of medicine, surgery, nursing, and anesthesia have all come such a long way in the past 20 years. Well-meaning individuals can unintentionally scare you with tales of their own surgeries, or a family member's surgery back in the 70's, 80's, and 90's!

That's the primary reason I decided to write this book. I wanted to give people the opportunity to learn how music affects the mind and the body and how to use music to allay their fears.

But this book is far more than information on music with surgery. It is intended to educate both the patient, as well as the clinician, on the extensive research that has been conducted in the last quarter century. I wanted more people to hear from patients who benefitted from using music to help ease their anxieties, their fears, their trepidations.

Music during the perioperative period – the time before, during, and after surgery – can benefit patients greatly in terms of reducing anxiety, decreasing pain perception, and improving outcomes.

While both planned surgery and unplanned surgery are stressful, unplanned surgery is often more stressful because you don't have time to process the new information. Your mind goes into overdrive with the increasing numbers of questions going unanswered, and the details of procedures you don't understand. The anxiety you feel emotionally triggers the body's reaction, which in turn responds by elevating heart rate, causing changes in breathing, and more. The sheer weight of the stress can become overwhelming.

On the other hand, a planned procedure can heighten anxiety due to the expanded time to worry. So why not take advantage of that extra time to help your mind and body handle the fear and anxiety in productive ways.

Music can be help alleviate the stress regardless of what triggered it.

CASE HISTORY 1: How Music Helped My Mother with Unplanned Bypass Surgery

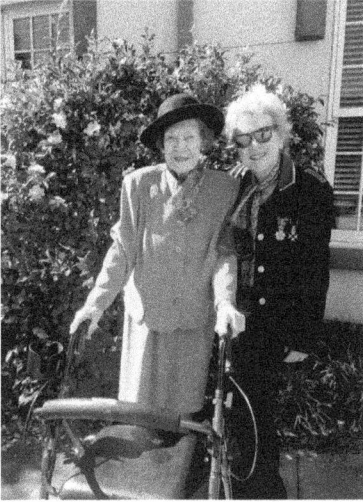

My mother learned unexpectedly that she needed heart by-pass surgery. She had no idea that she had a heart condition, even though her own father died of a massive heart attack at age 40 years old. At age 70, she attended a basketball game in a large university coliseum. During half-time, she headed to the ladies' room but struggled to going up the stairs without stopping every few rows to rest. It was the first time she had experienced this level of exhaustion when climbing stairs.

First Aid staff was summoned and arrived to check her out. They decided quickly to send her to the nearest hospital by ambulance. After a matter of hours there, doctors recommended sending her to a larger hospital for immediate heart bypass surgery.

Upon being notified, I grabbed some headphones and CDs, jumped into my car and made the long nine-hour drive to the hospital. At first, she wasn't sure that she wanted to wear headphones during surgery, but after I shared some of the medical research on the powerful benefits of listening to music before, during and after surgery, she agreed to try them. To my relief (this was 1996), her surgeon went along with my suggestion. He was optimistic, saying that it sounded like a very good idea.

At the time, I had not yet put together my proprietary playlist, so I began playing different CDs for her. After listening to several different tracks, Mother finally said, "Just play the music that *YOU* think would be best for me, as long as it's not *Nearer My God to Thee!*" We shared a hearty laugh. I chose George Frideric Handel's *Water Music* for her to listen to during surgery.

My father and I said a loving good-bye to my mother the morning of her bypass surgery, knowing the situation was extremely serious and she might not come through it. For five long hours we waited and worried. Suddenly, her young surgeon burst through the doors with a big smile on his face. He said she had come through the *five*-bypass operation with flying colors, was awakening in the recovery room, and asking to see us.

Normally, after surgery, my mother is extremely nauseated and disoriented. This time, it was unbelievably different. As we approached her bed in the recovery room, she began smiling and raised herself up just a little on her elbow. She said, "Oh Alice, the music was just beautiful!" Then she hummed a few bars of Handel's *Water Music*. I couldn't believe my eyes...or ears...because this experience was so very different from all her previous surgeries. Later, when she was back in her hospital room, she said, "I will never have surgery again without music through headphones! It made SUCH a difference!"

Mother also pointed out that in the recovery room the patients are separated only by curtains. Had she not been provided the headphones, she would have heard the other patients nearby moaning and crying out for the nurses. She said that the headphones blocked all of this out and she could just lie still and know that the surgery was over. Ever since then she reminds me to please tell everybody to use music through headphones when they have surgery.

This story and others, plus more information, are available throughout this book and on the Surgical Serenity Solutions website. Here's the link: https://www.surgicalserenitysolutions.com/video-testimonials

Stuff Happens When You Least Expect It

This is how it often happens. You're having a great day. You think you're in excellent health. Then, out of the blue, you're told you need emergency surgery. Learning beforehand about easy things you can do to help relieve the stress and uncertainty such situations generate can go a long way towards minimizing anxiety and helping the mind and body deal with things with more calmly. You won't be as prone to panic, thereby feeling more grounded and peaceful.

Not only have many surgical procedures today come a long way, many are safer and less invasive, often, requiring only tiny incisions.

The Washington Post published an interesting article about many of the advances in heart surgery on its website February 25, 2018. It provided a much brighter picture for those facing heart surgery in general, and for bypass surgery in particular, than was possible in years past.

It's worth reading. Here's a direct link to that article, *Once Scary, heart bypass surgery has become common and safer*:

www.washingtonpost.com/national/health-science/once-scary-heart-bypass-surgery-has-become-common-and-safer/2018/02/23/4b7459a4-157f-11e8-8b08-027a6ccb38eb_story.html

Technology Improvements and Specialists

In addition to dramatic improvements in surgical procedures, there are a growing number of specialists today. If you live in or near a large city, chances are excellent that you can find a surgeon for your specific procedure who has performed the surgery hundreds or thousands of times. Even hospitals and clinics in smaller and rural communities are working with a wide variety of specialists to offer local patients access to modern medical improvements right in their home communities.

These advances provide a certain level of reassurance to those with a tendency to worry and fret. However, even with continuing improvements in modern medical treatments and recovery, risk still exists. There will always be patients who struggle to cope. And if you're one of them,

Music to the Rescue

It's hard for me to imagine why anyone these days would not want to use music to calm their anxiety before a surgical or delicate procedure. I've witnessed the peace and tranquility and quicker recovery it brings to so many patients.

For those who do want to use music, Surgical Serenity Solutions provides the opportunity for you to either put together your own playlist or choose one of our carefully curated and sequenced playlists that were created specifically to improve surgical outcomes. The Surgical Serenity playlists have been tested on hundreds of patients and proven to calm and soothe in a powerful and safe manner. They actually have the power of stabilize blood pressure, heartbeat, and slow down the rapid, shallow breathing that creates more anxiety and prevents the blood from being as oxygenated as it should be. That's why they put the little monitor on your finger to check blood oxygen levels. When you're wearing your Serenity headphones, you'll be calm and relaxed!

CASE HISTORY 2: Planned knee replacement surgery

Elizabeth is a 55-year-old woman who had known for many months that she was going to need a knee replacement. She tried to avoid surgery, but the pain became too great. Reluctantly, she finally agreed to replacement surgery.

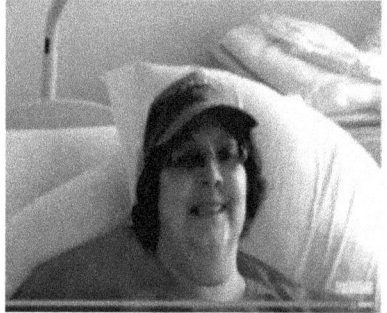

About a month before surgery, Elizabeth explained to me that she had had quite a few surgeries in the past, but that this one was in her words, "… really freaking her out!" She wasn't sure why the anxiety was so high this time, but she had read about our pre-loaded headphones and soothing music and definitely wanted to give them a try.

I think it's so interesting how she explained that once she had the headphones on and the music playing, she felt *more like an observer when they brought her into the operating room.* She explained how it felt like she was just watching a movie, and that after wearing the headphones throughout the surgery, she woke up feeling calm and oriented. This was totally unlike previous surgeries where she awoke feeling confused and disoriented.

Sometimes it's hard even for me to believe that something so simple as soothing music through headphones can make such a difference, but from the moment I started working with surgical patients using music through headphones, not one person has said that either it made no difference or that they wouldn't do it again!

I'm thrilled beyond measure to have helped so many relieve so much stress and anxiety.

See our website to learn more about our headphones and how to download our proprietary music playlists. Here's the link:
www.surgicalserenitysolutions.com/buyanapp

Take Your Own Kind of Music

Today, most doctors and hospitals will allow you to bring either your own music to listen to with headphones or earbuds, or they will allow pre-loaded headphones created especially for use before, during, and after surgery. Surgical Serenity Solutions' mobile app with five streaming surgical/medical playlists is currently available for individuals and organizations to download.

Pre-programmed, multi-headphone kits specifically designed for use in hospitals and clinics, and by medical professionals is currently available direct from Surgical Serenity Solutions on a limited basis. Updated kits are in development, as are additional music playlists.

What About Your Hospital?

Will **you** be allowed to bring headphones and music into the hospital operating room?

I wish I could give you an affirmative Yes! Unfortunately, while many hospitals have policies in place addressing this issue, many others at this time do not.

As evidenced throughout this book, most hospitals will allow a patient to bring our Surgical Serenity Solutions headphones into the entire perioperative area, but some will not allow a patient to bring anything from home into the operating or procedure room. However, with each passing day, new research studies are released containing empirical data regarding the benefits of music in the hospital, surgery center, or dental office. Some hospitals are taking the lead and introducing the use of music and headphones to patients themselves. Others are waiting to see how the trend progresses and may table any management decision on the idea until patients start pressing the issue.

This is why you want to bring up the question at your next pre-surgical visit. On the following page is a checklist of questions to ask your doctor or medical staff. Be aware that some doctors or nurses may defer the question to the anesthesiologist whom you may not meet until day of surgery. My research indicates that a vast majority *will* allow headphones and music *if* you can assure that the unit you intend to use are either brand new or intended specifically for surgery. The main question seems to be how it will be delivered to the patient and how much choice of music will the patient have.

Note: Some hospitals illegally use music streaming services like Pandora, Spotify, or others. The reason these are often illegal is that the hospitals use a private license and the terms of use don't allow sharing the music with others. Of course, the music from these services is NOT specially chosen to engage rhythmic entrainment or to reduce anxiety and improve surgical outcomes.

The Music Modernization Act of 2019 requires all healthcare facilities to purchase a license for any music that they play. Using Pandora, Spotify, or Apple Family Sharing without a healthcare license is illegal and will result in a fine that is considerably more than a license would be!

New research on the benefits of surgery with music comes out regularly, and as physicians read and hear more about this, more hospitals are opening up to the idea. I believe having hospitals purchase or provide headphones and music specially designed for surgery directly to patients is a good investment for them to consider. So, feel free to bring it to their attention.

Here's what I do know for certain: You have nothing to lose and everything to gain by asking permission to keep your headphones on throughout your surgery and in the recovery room.

CASE HISTORY 3: Using Musical Headphones without Prior Permission

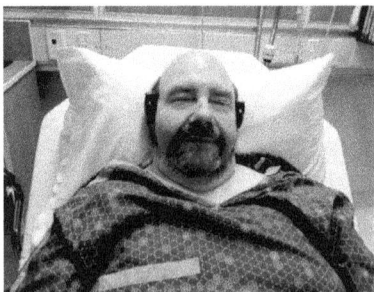

Here's how one new user in rural Michigan handled the situation when he went in for a pacemaker generator update. Dennis (his real name) didn't have the headphones yet when he already had his pre-surgery office visit so there was no opportunity to discuss using them with the surgeon.

Concerned how to adequately explain the purpose of using the cordless headphones and special music over the phone, Dennis and his wife decided to wait to ask until he was admitted and going through the initial pre-surgery procedure before broaching the subject with medical staff.

Once settled into his room and bed, Dennis put on his headphones and settled back to listen and relax. His wife sat nearby reading a book.

Several nurses and technicians came by to verify paperwork, check vitals, and set up IVs. Dennis continued wearing the headphones expecting someone to ask about them, but no one did. Eventually, his assigned nurse came in again to check the drip and said he'd be headed to the surgical suite on time within the next 20 minutes or so.

It was then that Dennis' wife pulled the Surgical Serenity Solutions headphone's box out of her bag and handed it to the nurse. While the nurse read the information on the box, the wife explained those were the headphones Dennis was wearing. She then asked if the nurse thought there would be any problem with him wearing them during the procedure. The nurse wasn't sure but said she'd check, and just before heading out of the room turned and added, "Those sound really interesting. I think I could use a set to relax with on break."

The nurse never came back with an answer. However, a surgical technician came by a minutes later to discuss final details. She was also shown the product box and asked if Dennis could wear them into surgery. The technician said she didn't see a problem and rolled Dennis off to surgery. He was still wearing them a couple hours later when they returned him to his room.

Dennis said no one questioned why he was wearing headphones. He didn't know if the technician had gotten the doctor's or anesthesiologist's permission or not.

While the classical music track wasn't his favorite genre, and a bit annoying when he first put on the headphones, by the time he was out of recovery he'd grown comfortable with the selections. He continued wearing them until discharged an hour earlier than predicted, during the ride home, and off and on for several days during recuperation. He's looking forward to trying out the Jazz playlist for his next procedure.

See our website to learn more about our headphones and how to download our proprietary music playlists. Here's the link:
www.surgicalserenitysolutions.com/buyanapp

CHECKLIST: Questions to Ask Your Doctor Before Surgery

1. Will I be allowed to take music and my own headphones into surgery?

2. If not, will I be allowed to take Surgical Serenity Solutions pre-loaded, cordless headphones into surgery? (Cleveland Clinic, Mayo Clinic, Johns Hopkins and other facilities already allow patients to have headphones that are pre-loaded.)

3. If not, will the hospital provide streaming music just intended to calm the patient, through Bluetooth headphones, Bluetooth earbuds, AirPods, or similar ear plug devices?

4. During the surgery, will you allow the music to keep playing continuously?

Numerous research studies show that even though I may not be consciously hearing it, my body will still respond to the slow, steady pulse, and the music will greatly muffle other music that might be playing in the operating room, as well as block out conversations that could be potentially upsetting to me.

The Surgical Serenity Solutions website contains many articles and links to authoritative research studies: www.surgicalserenitysolutions.com/medical-research/

The Journal of Clinical Oncology website includes a comprehensive report from October 1, 2015, on the "Effects of Music Therapy on Anesthesia Requirements and Anxiety in Women Undergoing Ambulatory Breast Surgery for Cancer

Diagnosis and Treatment: A Randomized Controlled Trial".
See the report here:
www.ncbi.nlm.nih.gov/pmc/articles/PMC4979095/

You can download a printable copy of this checklist from our website.
https://www.surgicalserenitysolutions.com/free-

CHAPTER 2
Continuing Your Recovery at Home with Music

After your surgery is over and you've been discharged, you'll be going home to rest and recuperate. This is a time when your music can be as calming, soothing, and beneficial as ever. Immediately after surgery, there is a sense of relief that the problem has been remedied and that you will soon be "good as new" and back to your life, better than ever. But it really is important not to overdo it or try to return to your regular routine too soon.

The hospital and doctor will undoubtedly offer pain medication but remember that the power of music to block pain perception is well-documented. The more that you can relax to music through headphones, the less pain medication you will likely need.

This is a potentially dangerous time when patients believe they need more pain medication than they really do. Inadvertently, they can become dependent on their pain medication. When initial supplies run out and they are craving more, they may or may not realize that they have become addicted to their pain medication. As I mentioned elsewhere, the opioid crisis is raging around the world. To my knowledge no country or state has escaped its ravages.

No one initially intends to take pain medication to excess, but each of us has different pain thresholds. Some need more medication than others to manage their pain level. When the prescribed medication runs out and no more refills are allowed, people, overwhelmed with a sense of desperation, some people look on the streets to find someone who will sell them anything to ease their pain.

Next steps after Your Procedure

When you're leaving the hospital, clinic, or surgery center, be sure to pack up your headphones to take home with you. If the doctor provided headphones that belong to the hospital, of course you'll want to have some waiting for you at home. Once your surgery is over, you'll either recuperate for a few more days in the hospital or you'll be going home to your own familiar environment and comforts of home. Be sure to take your music and headphones with you into the recuperation stage.

By now, this music will be familiar to you and will hopefully be associated with feelings of safety, comfort, and security. That's the beauty of "conditioning." Our proprietary playlists have music that has been either created or carefully chosen for its ability to calm the body and the mind. This process has even been patented so that other creators of relaxing music can't claim that it works as well for surgery. Once you're well past this period of convalescence, you can think about going back to your own preferred music, which is probably more upbeat and more complex. In other words, you'll have music with lyrics, more varied instruments and greater musical and rhythmic variety in general.

Before you know it, your surgery will be a dim memory that is fading into the past, and you'll be feeling so much better than you did before. I believe that we are intended to enjoy our lives, do the work we best know how to do and have enthusiasm for, and help others as we can.

The Surgical Serenity Solutions App is now available for iPhone, iTouch, and Android devices. The following playlists are featured:

- Classical Blend

- Jazz

- New Age

- Lullabies

- Memory Care

Users can select one or multiple playlists. Playlists are designed for continuous play throughout the procedure, regardless of length.

We recommend that patients listen to playlists using earbuds or headphones so that extraneous noise and conversations are eliminated.

Visit the Surgical Serenity Solutions website for direct links to purchase the app of your choice. Click here or type this URL into your device browser:
www.surgicalserenitysolutions.com/digital-products/

Confused about which playlist would be best for you?

The next chapter will provide some interesting perspective to help you understand the best type of music to use during surgery. Plus, you'll discover why just listening to your absolute favorite music is not always the best choice.

CHAPTER 3

What Is the Best Type of Music to Use During Surgery?

Since the mid- 1980's neuroscientists and social scientists have been seriously studying and researching the mind-body connection. There's absolutely no doubt that emotions powerfully affect the body and music elicits every possible human emotion. Music is also powerfully connected to memories and associations.

Individuals can have very differing associations with different pieces of music, so I recommend choosing music for yourself that is not familiar specifically, but is in a genre that you know you like, such as classical, jazz, New Age or lullabies. You don't know what associations or emotions will be triggered by specific pieces which is why unfamiliar pieces work best.

If you can naturally relax and calm your body and mind before surgery through music, research shows that you can get a better outcome, such as healing faster and requiring less medication, including anxiety meds, (usually benzodiazepines) the actual anesthesia or sedative drug, and pain medication.

Instead of worrying about the quality of the surgery, you can reduce your anxiety level—because it affects your recovery. Anxiety also affects how you feel, obviously, but most people don't realize that anxiety affects recovery time and quality.

"Dr. Cash, thank you so much for helping me choose the perfect music for my hip replacement surgery. The procedure went exceptionally smoothly and knowing that I had music that I loved made everything easier. I plan to be back on my cross-country skis in February." – Barb E., patient

More and more, doctors are becoming aware of the power of music to calm and comfort the patient naturally, reduce anxiety, and get them home and back to their lives faster. A quick Google search of "Surgery with Music" will bring you dozens of clinical studies, medical journal articles, magazine articles, and news clips from the major networks that document the benefits of music before, during, and after the operation (called the perioperative period). In fact, the calmer you are, the less medication you will likely need, and the less medication you require, the fewer side-effects you'll risk, and the faster you will recover and get back to your life. I have links to some of these studies in Chapter 15.

Because the doctors often listen to their own music, (which isn't chosen to be relaxing for the patient,) the music for patients works best when listened to through headphones or earbuds.

Knowing that may not alleviate your fear, however just gathering information like this can be helpful and reassuring.

Articles on music and surgery come to my email multiple times per week, so I know both physicians and patients are learning about it. The increase in studies on music with surgery has increased 100% in the last decade so we know that our society is ready to look at non-chemical methods for calming patients, decreasing pain perception, while increasing patient satisfaction.

"My son's surgery was yesterday. He wore the headset for two hours before surgery and during the procedure. Unlike his last surgery, all went well. Lots of people were involved to make sure he reacted well to the anesthesia and other medicines provided. They were very happy to let him use the headphones in the operating room. He went into surgery thinking the headset would

be helpful in keeping him calm and needing less anesthesia, and he did remain calm after coming around post-op. We believe your music was integral to his good experience. Many thanks!" – Faith Nuygen, mother of patient

How Music Calms Anxiety

The power of music to calm anxiety, lift depression, inspire ideas and behavior changes, and process grief is well-known. But how does music do this? Music permeates all aspects of our culture. Every car that has been built for the past 80 years has, at the very least, a radio. We've seen the addition of FM radio, cassette players, CD players, multi-CD players, Bluetooth connections to our devices, and Sirius satellite radio. It really is quite remarkable. Almost everyone on the planet has some kind of music that they really love.

Why do people want music in almost every place that they go? One reason is it energizes them and takes them away from the uncomfortable emotions they may be feeling. When road rage suddenly erupts, calming music can help. In the movie *"The Shawshank Redemption,"* when the prisoners were in their walled and barbed-wire exercise yard, classical music was suddenly broadcast through huge outdoor speakers and the prisoners almost immediately became calm and soon were slowly walking around calmly and peacefully.

When people hear beautiful anthems or solos in a spiritual or sacred setting, or when the congregation sings hymns and responses in church, they feel uplifted and are often moved to tears. Listening to the words from the Bible and other holy books set to music is a powerful part of the worship experience. Music in a religious or spiritual setting can inspire people to change for the better and motivate them to do all kinds of productive things. Music is powerful in more ways than most people ever realize.

Characteristics of the ideal music

What is the ideal type of music for surgery — before, during and after?

For most people, music is a pleasant force in their lives. We have music wherever we go, our homes, our cars, restaurants, airplanes, cruise ships. Nearly everywhere!

But in our society, music is taken for granted. It is often used to set a mood, to distract, or to obscure an unpleasant sound. But how much thought or study is really put into it? We all know about the mindless "elevator music" or even worse, the "on-hold" music that companies play when we are forced to wait for the next customer-service or reservation agent.

As a professional musician, I find some of the music quite offensive and even intolerable, but every now and then, I actually hear something I enjoy and that puts me in a good mood! Being aware of the type of music you are listening to, and why you like or dislike something in particular is a very good way to surround yourself with music that makes you feel most calm, secure, and happy.

Music does affect the mind, the body, and the spirit. There's no question about that. And it is an individual matter. It affects the mind because of all the associations we have with music. It doesn't even have to be a specific type of music but let's say you respond well to orchestral, classical music. Perhaps you grew up playing the violin and your parents took you to orchestra concerts. You grew up knowing the music of Bach,

Mozart and Tchaikovsky and feel happy and secure when you hear this music.

Or perhaps you grew up hearing jazz in your home and took up playing the saxophone or the string bass when you were old enough. When you hear jazz music, you feel happy, calm and secure. Familiar music produces familiar responses of calm and peacefulness.

But, let's say that you had a negative experience with a specific piece of music. One that you now dislike for whatever reason, whether you played it, heard it, or just have a negative association with it. There are many pieces of music that some people love, and others dislike intensely because it has a negative association for them personally.

I had a very negative reaction to a pop song that came out in summer of 1975 because I was pregnant and did not realize it that at the time. Now, many years later, I can hear that song and I still feel nauseated and sick within seconds. Music is that powerful.

For these reasons, the right kind of music for surgery may vary from individual to individual. However, I do recommend that music for surgery be offered:

- in a variety of genres so that people can listen to a genre they like

- using pieces of music that are not particularly familiar to most people, so that there's little chance of eliciting a negative association

Music is very personal and musical taste varies greatly. So, when I'm choosing music of a specific genre that will appeal to lots of people, I choose music of that genre that is relatively unfamiliar.

Music affects the mind, body and spirit no matter the genre, but the power of rhythmic entrainment can be harnessed in any genre of music. I explain rhythmic entrainment after the next two case histories.

Finding the Best Type of Music for You to Use During Surgery

To understand how to choose the best music for your surgical/dental procedure, it is helpful to understand the basic components of music in general. Here are the building blocks of music:

- Melody: the "tune" or single-line melody

- Harmony: multiple strands of music that blend together

- Rhythm: the long and short-note combinations that create a steady beat or a more varied beat.

- Tempo: the speed of the music

- Timbre: the overall tone quality of the music, based on which instruments are used.

There are other things to be considered in choosing music for therapeutic purposes, but the above items are part of ALL music. These components have evolved through the millennia and music is always in a state of flux. However, it's clear that music is very personal for people and is often tied to strong memories. For that reason, the music I have chosen for Surgical Serenity Solutions is not familiar specifically, but the various genres will *feel* familiar to you.

No one is going to dictate to you what music you must use during surgery, and I think that's very important for you to know in advance that you will be given a choice. But it's also very important for you to know what research shows the basic characteristics of the ideal music for surgery are.

Most Important Characteristic about the Music You Use

The **most important** characteristic for your music during surgery is that the music be **slow, steady, and soothing**, so that it engages **rhythmic entrainment** and induces a physiological state akin to the "relaxation response."

CASE HISTORY 4: Caesarian section with Highly Anxious Mother

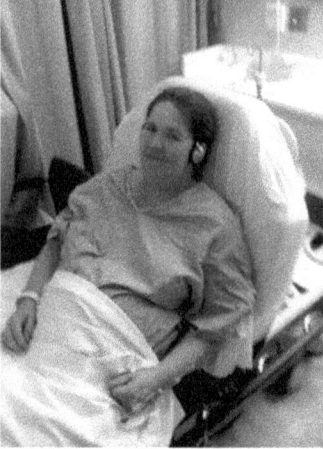

In 2010, this 34-year old first-time mother was told that she would have to have her baby by Caesarean section because of a fibroid tumor that was blocking the birth canal. She was not planning to have the baby this way and was not pleased to know that she really had no choice.

Because this patient was also a professional musician and had heard about the benefits of music in the perioperative period, she acquired some of Surgical Serenity Solutions' pre-loaded headphones and listened for the hour after she was prepped, but before she was taken back for the actual Caesarean section. She later told me that the headphones were a lifesaver before the surgery because she was separated only by a curtain from the dozen or so other women scheduled that day. She said that many of them were upset and berating their husbands or significant others for various reasons and that having the classical music playing through headphones kept her calm and blocked "about 95%" of the chaos in the pre-op area. When you're in the pre-op area, waiting to be taken into your procedure, you don't want to hear the other patients around you talking about what they are going through, because it is often unpleasant conversation.

How Long Will You Need to Wait?

The all too common experience of noisy chaos during the pre-op period is why using music *before* a procedure, as well as during and after is so very helpful!

Sometimes I have patients say, "but the procedure doesn't take but 10 minutes," referring to some eye surgeries or small procedures. The problem is that you have no idea how long you'll be waiting in pre-op with just a curtain separating you from other anxious patients who don't have the benefit of soothing music. The surgeon may give you an ideal timetable for how long you'll be in each stage of the procedure, but emergencies happen all the time and if you are prepared with your soothing music, you will be so happy that you thought and planned ahead.

CASE HISTORY 5: Patient with Multiple, Consecutive Surgeries

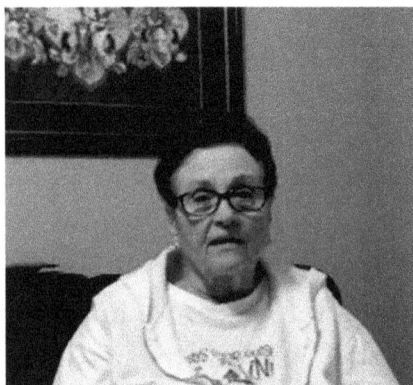

This 70-year old patient had no history of health issues or any surgery at all. She had been feeling just a little tired for a few days and suddenly had a very serious heart attack. She was rushed to the local hospital and had emergency surgery to put stents in her heart that would allow the blood to flow easier. After the surgery, medical staff had a very difficult time waking her back up and finally had to use Narcan, the drug that is administered to people who have overdosed on drugs. This was very terrifying to this patient. She did begin to recover, unfortunately, five days after she returned home, she suffered a ruptured appendix!

She was rushed to the hospital and underwent surgery, this time without the benefit of music or headphones. Again, she was recovering from her surgeries at home but now with tremendous anxiety and pain, and on top of that she began developing serious insomnia due to the stress.

She read online about the power of soothing music through headphones. She acquired some of our headphones and was just beginning to listen when her doctor called and told her that she needed to have surgery again to implant a pacemaker and a defibrillator.

The patient contacted me and asked about coping with her intense anxiety about the procedure and her fears of not being able to awaken from anesthesia since that had happened just a few weeks previously. We talked at length about lying down every afternoon for at least 30 minutes and listening to the music with her eyes closed to practice engaging rhythmic entrainment. By the time her pacemaker and defibrillator implantation were scheduled, she felt she was prepared to go in and use the music to calm her before the procedure and to help her wake up after. She happily reported that was exactly what happened.

To hear this patient tell her story, click here or type into your browser:
www.surgicalserenitysolutions.com/video-testimonals/#heart-attack-appendicitis-defibrillator-implant

CASE HISTORY 6: Using Music for Pacemaker Implantation

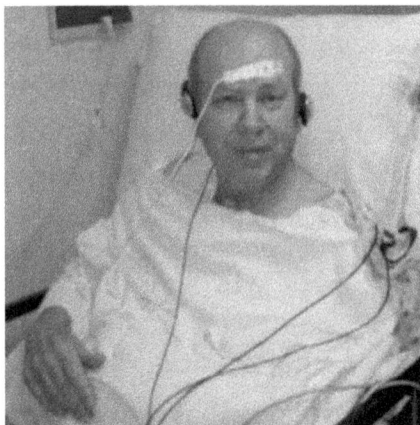

This patient, John H., reported proudly that he never went to the doctor growing up. He believed that if he ate fresh, farm-grown food and spent lots of time outdoors, he would naturally stay healthy. Everything was going well until he had a massive heart-attack at age 55.

When I met this patient, he was 10 years post heart-attack and had also been diagnosed with Parkinson's disease. Now he was being told he needed a pacemaker and was not looking forward to it. Here is a picture of him on the day of his procedure, wearing his surgical headphones, pre-loaded with soothing music.

After the procedure he explained that when he arrived at the hospital the morning of the surgery, he was full of fear and anxiety. He had never had anesthesia before and wasn't sure how he would react to it. His body temperature was well below normal and his blood pressure had dropped to 70/40. He said that he felt "really bad" and they were considering postponing the procedure. Then he remembered that he had brought his "surgery headphones" and asked his wife to put them on him.

After his procedure, he became what we call a "true believer" and extolled the power of the "right" music through headphones to everyone he met. He always wanted me to create a country music playlist, but to this day, I can't think of enough country music that would be appropriate to listen as you're going into or coming out of surgery. Suggestions welcomed!

In a follow-up video testimonial John sent to me, he shared that in less than 15 minutes once he put on the headphones and began listening to the calming music, his body began warming up and his blood pressure had stabilized. It was soon good enough for him to proceed with the pacemaker implantation as scheduled.

John had a normal and uneventful recovery. He believes that the music through headphones made a huge difference for him. His doctors had told him that the procedure could take up to six hours because of his serious heart problem and the amount of medication they would have to use.

When John woke up in the recovery area, he said that the first thing he noticed was that the music was still playing and that it was very reassuring because he knew instantly that he had survived it and had been "given another chance at life." He said that he was up and walking after four hours and that he went home the next morning with only Tylenol for pain.

To listen to him tell this powerful story himself click here or type into your browser: www.surgicalserenitysolutions.com/heart

---

Note the Effects of Using Slow, Steady, Purely Instrumental Music

This is the kind of result that I hear frequently after patients use the right kind of slow, steady, purely instrumental music for their surgical procedure.

CASE HISTORY 7: Macular Hole Surgery

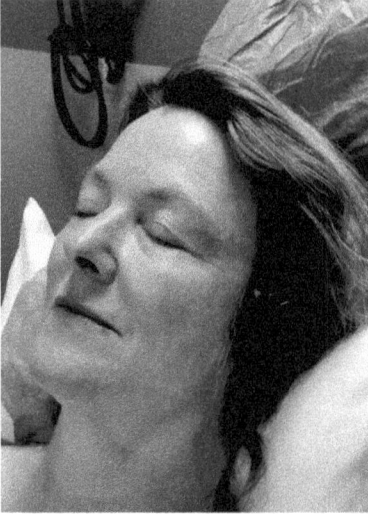

This woman has always taken good care of herself, gone for physicals and exercised. Recently, she went to her eye doctor for a routine examination and found that she had developed a "Macular hole" that required immediate surgery. She was quite disconcerted by this and baffled by how it could have happened. But that's how life is sometimes, you think you're doing all the right things, and then something pops up out of the blue that requires surgery. Because she is a good friend, I offered her some of my pre-programmed serenity headphones and she gladly accepted. She was told that she needed the surgery within 5 days or the hole could expand and permanently affect her vision.

Once she received the headphones, she spent 30-60 minutes per day lying on the couch and relaxing to the soothing, rhythmic, classical music and by the day of the surgery, just 3 days later, she was conditioned to relaxing physically and emotionally when she heard this music.

The day of the surgery arrived, and she put the headphones on while waiting to be called back for the prep. This is the patient after she has been prepped, listening to the soothing music, pre-surgery. "Before they called me back, I was sitting in a crowded waiting room, filled with people who all seemed to be anxious about their procedures. The air was filled with negative, gloomy conversations and I had nowhere to go. Even the TV was blaring out negative news. I felt trapped and a little panicky, but my eye doctor had said that I needed the eye surgery immediately or my sight in that eye could be jeopardized forever."

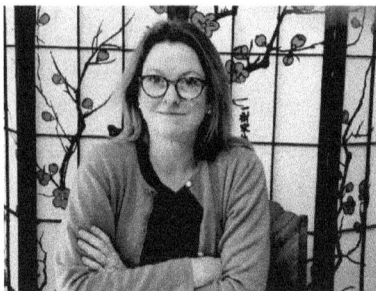

[Photo of same woman, Case History #8]

"I was actually holding your headphones in their box, waiting to put them on after they called me back. Then my friend said, 'why don't you put on the headphones now?' I put on my surgical headphones and that was the beginning of relief and a feeling of being transported to another, more tranquil world. I can't begin to tell you how grateful I am for this amazing device and it's soothing music."

To hear her tell the story, click or type in https://www.surgicalserenitysolutions.com/eyes

She explained to me afterwards that the anxiety-reducing power of this music through headphones, allowed her to calm down enough that she did not need any anxiety medication before or after the procedure.

After she returned home she had a complicated post-surgical experience because she had to keep her head (and eyes) completely immobilized, but with the help of her soothing and calming playlist, and access to new soothing playlists in other styles, she got through it with no further damage to eyes.

CHAPTER 4

Benefits of Using Music Before, During, and After Surgery

The "perioperative period" is simply the time beginning immediately before the surgery or procedure (preoperative) and ending with the recovery (postoperative) period, when patient has arrived at the hospital and is either waiting to be checked in, or has been checked in and is waiting to be taken to pre-op, where they change into a gown, get their IV started and wait patiently for surgery to begin.

Let's discuss the value of music during all three phases.

Music During the Preoperative Phase

The preoperative phase starts when patient arrives at the hospital and is waiting to be taken to pre-op, to change into a gown, get the IV started and wait for surgery to begin.

Often, when patients have their headphones and music, they do not need any anxiety medication before their procedure because the music is relaxing them and keeping them relaxed. This is ideal because when they're ready to be taken to the operating room, they are calm but alert and the surgeon or anesthesiologist can talk with them about what's going to be happening.

Here are some patients I've worked with wearing their pre-loaded headphones during the pre-operative period:

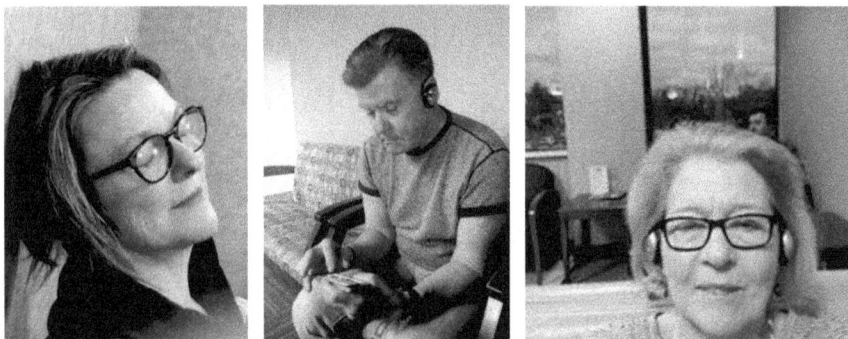

Once you've been prepped for surgery and wheeled down to the operating room, it's important to keep the headphones on as you're being either put to sleep or put into a calm state with a sedative (such as Versed/midazolam), as well as given some pain medication. While you're wearing the headphones the slow, steady, calming music keeps your heartbeat and breathing stabilized because of rhythmic entrainment.

If you are under general anesthesia, you do cease to consciously hear the music, however because of the power of rhythmic entrainment, your body still responds to the slow, steady pulse or beat of the music. This is one of the most important aspects of music through headphones during surgery that many patients have not been aware of in the past. Even if you, personally, have never awakened from surgery remembering comments that weren't positive, it happens every day and is easy to prevent.

Also important is understanding that calming music through headphones blocks conversations of medical staff which can sometimes be quite upsetting and possibly negative. These conversations can stay in your subconscious and can cause more anxiety after the procedure.

You may encounter medical personnel who say there is no point in wearing these headphones throughout the surgery, but the fact is that even if they only blocked out the medical team's conversations, it would be a good idea. In the case of procedures that typically use regional anesthesia, or simply "sedation" drugs, the good thing is that if the doctor needs to ask you a question, you can still hear him or her asking you a question directly.

The fact that the music is continuing to play is even more of a benefit because the rhythmic entrainment is working on keeping your heartbeat and breathing stable during the procedure, plus the music is beautiful and calming while you lie there.

Music in the Recovery Room

This postoperative period is an extremely beneficial time to have the headphones on because you must stay in recovery until all nausea and vomiting has ceased. Often, the medical staff want you to be able to answer certain basic questions to their satisfaction, and this is important. Hospital and insurance companies have regulations about how long a patient must be nausea-free and awake before they may be discharged. While you're in the recovery area, the "meter is running" so that the sooner you can safely leave, the more your wallet will appreciate it!

Of course, all of your body rhythms need to have stabilized and the pain level must be manageable. For those that have had numerous surgeries and know that they are extremely susceptible to post-surgical nausea and vomiting, confusion, and agitation, having soothing music playing as you wake up can ease that reaction and help you to leave the recovery area sooner.

CASE HISTORY 8: Apprehension Regarding Anesthesia During Gall Bladder Surgery

One patient described her apprehension regarding being administered anesthesia during gall bladder surgery this way:

> *"In August 2014, I had gall bladder surgery. I was apprehensive since I was so slow to come out of the anesthesia during past surgeries. I never saw the inside of the recovery rooms. It took so long they just moved me on to the post-op room.*
>
> *For a future surgery I used the Surgical Serenity headphones for a couple of weeks prior to the surgery, plus before and during the surgery and recovery. Prior to the surgery, my blood pressure was lower than normal, and I woke up in the recovery room for the first time ever! I highly recommend these headphones to anyone preparing to have surgery!" – Mary Jo Linker*

Remember: A Patient Under Anesthesia Stops "Hearing the Music" but the Body Continues to Respond to the Music Vibrations

While the patient is under anesthesia, it's important to understand that he or she stops "hearing" the music, but the body still responds to the slow, steady pulse of the music and responds by staying entrained to the music.

The Surgical Serenity Solutions App is available for iPhone, iTouch, and Android devices. Five different playlists are available.

We recommend that patients listen to playlists using earbuds or headphones so that extraneous noise and conversations are eliminated.

Visit the Surgical Serenity Solutions website for direct links to purchase the app of your choice. Click here or type this URL into your device browser:
www.surgicalserenitysolutions.com/digital-products/

CHAPTER 5

Music with Dentistry and Other Medical Procedures

Can music make a difference in the dental chair? Of course! Nobody likes going to the dentist! The sound of the drill alone freaks some people out and makes them want to run away. Knowing that you're lying on your back and a man (usually) that you don't know very well is leaning over you, usually less than 12 inches from your face, is unnerving. Then there's the fact that pain can strike at any moment while the drilling and probing are taking place.

How does music help with that? As with other types of surgical or medical procedures, you begin listening to your favorite slow, soothing music while you're in the waiting room and by the time you're called into the dental procedure room, you're going to begin to drift into the relaxation response and muscle tension will relax, racing thoughts will slow down and you are likely to have a better experience.

Here's what one dental patient said:

"I had to have a series of painful dental procedures. For the first two, I did not have the Surgical Serenity headphones, but then I found out about them and got them immediately. What a difference! The first procedures, I sat in the chair completely tensed up and waiting for the pain. It was miserable! The last time, I used the headphones and actually relaxed and enjoyed listening to the beautiful, relaxing music. They are so comfortable and have no cords to interfere with dentist's machinery. I will recommend them to everyone." – Suzanne Bergmeister, PhD, MBA professor at University of Louisville, KY

Dentists were actually among the first to utilize the power of music during their procedures. In the 1950's they had big clunky headphones that fit over the top of the patient's head and they administered what they called "audio analgesia." We have many scientific studies and articles about the dentist's audio analgesia, but by the late 1970's, it seems that many dentists had forgotten about the importance of delivering the music through headphones and were installing TVs in the operatory, or simply a radio playing "easy listening" music on a shelf nearby. The whole point of delivering that music through headphones is to muffle the sound of the drill, while allowing patient to hear questions or instructions from the dentist.

Another one of our patients said:

> *"I had my dental surgery on with your surgery music and it was wonderful. I had begun listening to the music ahead of time, so they were like old friends when surgery time rolled around. I was calm and relaxed before surgery. The dentist and staff tucked me in, made sure I had my music, away we went. Post-op I was still relaxed – had a sleep and had little pain. I had a bunch of work done – I did take an Advil at bedtime just for "insurance" but really didn't need it."* – Ann Thoen from New Zealand

Simply because going to the dentist, even for a check-up and cleaning, is one of the most dreaded experiences, I encourage all dentists to have headphones and soothing music waiting for the patient. It's so simple and with Bluetooth headphones available now or pre-loaded, cordless headphones, there no worry about cords getting in the way of the dentist and his equipment.

I remember going to see my dentists in the '80's or '90's and suddenly he had TVs in the corner of the room as well as in the ceiling, but without headphones, I could still hear the drill way too much. Then at one point he got virtual reality goggles, but they too still didn't block the sound of the drill, tooth polisher and other machines. I do believe that most dental offices try their best to make their patients comfortable, but it's just not a happy procedure.

CASE HISTORY 9: Dental Patient with Series of Fillings, Crowns and Root Canal

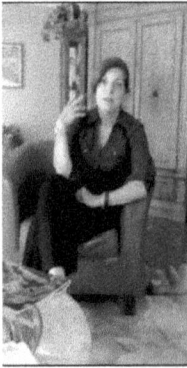

This 45-year-old woman was in the middle of a series of dental procedures, including a crown and some difficult fillings. She had already had two lengthy visits to the dentist when she heard about the power of music through headphones when going to the dentist.

She explained, "Several months ago I had a couple of fillings replaced and I did not have the headphones. I went in and it was the most unpleasant hour of my life because there was a lot of drilling and a lot of noise and a lot of anxiety on my part because I wasn't sure when it was going to hurt and when it wasn't going to hurt. That's all I could focus on ... when was the drilling was starting and when it was stopping.

"The next time I went back I had several more fillings replaced on the other side, plus I had a crown put in resulting in even more drilling. But this time I had the headphones on. Seriously, it made all the difference in the world because the music was very soothing. I could still hear the dentist when he had to ask me a question or tell me to spit or whatever. But I could concentrate more on the music rather than the drilling. I found myself relaxing and listening to the music because it was so pleasant.

I would absolutely recommend them. I haven't used them yet for anything besides the dental work but I can see the benefit no matter what [type of medical procedure] someone was going through. They really help keep your mind off whatever you're worried about."

To hear this patient tell her story, click type www.SurgicalSerenitySolutions.com/crown

---

For Best Results Use Headphones Before, During, and After Dental Procedures

Putting on the headphones while waiting to be called back is a very good idea because the slow, steady rhythms calm the anxious heart rate and rapid breathing. Once you're in the dental chair, the headphones will greatly help to muffle the sound of the drill while still allowing the dentist to ask necessary questions and give you instructions.

Knowing that the right music can also decrease pain perception, it's possible that you won't even need Novocain, nitrous oxide, or anything but music.

Patients with multiple, complicated conditions

Of course, every surgery and patient response is unique, but when patients have multiple issues going on at the same time, it can be a challenge for the doctors. Oftentimes, people who already have chronic medical issues like diabetes, heart disease, or hypertension have a new issue appear. For example, many pregnant women, who did not previously have high blood pressure or diabetes, develop these conditions during pregnancy. This is a perfect example of complex medical issues that must be dealt with both individually and as a cluster. Also, see https://www.SurgicalSerenitySolutions.com/dental

When I work with patients like this, I always suggest that calming, slow, steady music through headphones is the perfect non-chemical way to keep them calm during this period.

"My name is Mary Jo ... I am a female age 63. About 4 years ago I was diagnosed with SSNHL, which is a sudden sensorineural hearing loss. I was also diagnosed with severe hyperacusis and severe tinnitus. I have been under anesthesia 3 times since then, and the noise in my head has gotten louder each time following the surgery. I will also mention I do not do well with anesthesia......nausea and vomiting and usually wake up crying and very disoriented... I wore the headphones about 40 minutes a day the week before the knee surgery to get used to them. The classical piano WAS NOT hard to get used to!!! It was wonderful. The morning of surgery I put the headphones on before being taken back. I woke up much calmer, absolutely no nausea or vomiting then or at home, and my ears do not seem to be any worse this time. I thank God for Dr. Cash. I think she has developed a product that can help so many people!" – Mary Jo

Screening Procedures

Another challenge for patients is the screening procedures like mammograms and colonoscopies when we reach a certain age. Many procedures such as mammograms and colonoscopies are not covered by insurance unless there are clear symptoms indicating that there might be a problem. As we get older, the screening procedures become very important and many colon polyps, cysts in the breasts, and beginning cataracts are caught early. But these procedures can be painful and cause anxiety, just because you're anticipating pain. Music through headphones is a proven way to get through these procedures.

CASE HISTORY 10: First Colonoscopy Screening

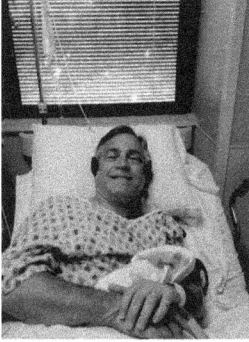

This patient told me that since he had just turned 50, he had been told that he would need a routine screening colonoscopy. He was not looking forward to it but said that he was aware that listening to calming music through headphones could really make a difference as he went through the process. He ordered the pre-loaded headphones about a week in advance and spent about 30 minutes each day listening to the calming music while lying down.

On the day of the procedure, he put his headphones on as soon as he checked in at hospital and went right into his state of relaxation and entrainment. Afterwards he said that it was not nearly as bad as he had anticipated. This is what happens 99 percent of the time!

To hear his story, click here or type into your browser: https://www.surgicalserenitysolutions.com/colon

The Surgical Serenity Solutions App is available for iPhone, iTouch, and Android devices.

Users can select one or multiple playlists. Playlists are designed for continuous play throughout the procedure, regardless of length.

We recommend that patients listen to playlists using earbuds or headphones so that extraneous noise and conversations are eliminated.

Visit the Surgical Serenity Solutions website for direct links to purchase the app of your choice. Click here or type this URL into your device browser:

www.surgicalserenitysolutions.com/digital-products/

CHAPTER 6

Music and the Mind-Body Connection

In this chapter, you'll learn more about how music affects the body, both physically and emotionally, as well as the differences between music therapy and music medicine, and read two more case histories.

How music affects you physically and emotionally

We all know intuitively that music affects our moods and our emotions, but it also affects our physical bodies through a process called rhythmic entrainment. We'll talk more about that soon. When music with a strong rhythm is playing, it's almost impossible not to get up and move to it, clap your hands, or tap your toes! It's absolutely impossible to separate the mind and the body but we know that music affects us at an energetic, cellular level, and brings back happy and sad feelings and memories. There is no doubt that music can fill you with energy or slow you down so that you can breathe easier and relax. The fields of music therapy, music medicine, sound healing, and vibrational healing exist to help us all create better health and better lives through music and sound. This definitely applies to surgery and preparing for surgery.

People who are not professional music healers or sound healers find creative ways to use music in their lives. I had a patient once who was an executive in a large company. He had a long drive to work in the mornings and related to me that he had just bought a new car that had a six-CD changer in it and to make his drive easier, he "programmed" his morning commute with music. When he left home in the morning he was listening to soothing, favorite jazz standards, moving to Top 40s midway through, and by the time he drove into the parking lot of his office building, the music playing was the theme to "Superman!" What a great idea!

All this is to say that music really can energize one's body and mind. And before surgery, it can calm and comfort, as well as stabilize body rhythms.

Ever since the early 1990's neuro-scientists and social scientists have been seriously studying and researching the mind-body connection. There's absolutely no doubt that emotions powerfully affect the body and music elicits every possible human emotion. Music is also powerfully connected to memories and associations. Because people can have very differing associations with different pieces of music, for surgery, I recommend choosing music for yourself that is not familiar specifically, but is in a genre that you know you like, such as classical, jazz, New Age or lullabies. You don't know what associations or emotions will be triggered by specific pieces which is why unfamiliar pieces work best.

Remember, if you can naturally relax and calm your body and mind before surgery through music, research shows that you will get a better result, heal faster, and require less medication.

The Difference between Music Therapy and Music Medicine

Around the world, music is being used for therapeutic purposes by healthcare professionals who have a variety of different kinds of training. Sometimes it is nurses, sometimes it's chaplains, sometimes it's surgeons or anesthesiologists who are offering music through headphones. The beauty is that that music has proven to be therapeutic and beneficial to patients who are have surgery or other medical/dental procedures that are anxiety provoking.

Sometimes it is being offered by an actual music therapist who has gone to school to study music therapy and done a supervised internship in a clinical setting. Music therapists are quite skilled and can accomplish many therapeutic goals through music. But music therapy, technically only happens when a music therapist is present and has assessed the patient's needs and strengths. They have also created a relationship with the patient. This is a highly desirable goal, but unfortunately, there are far more patients having surgery, dental work, joint replacements and kidney dialysis than there are music therapists. Plus, in these days of cutbacks all over the hospital and healthcare environments, hospitals are usually not willing to hire more than three or four music therapists. A large hospital might have a dozen, but they are certainly not all there all the time.

Also, music therapists tend to work in more of a rehabilitation setting. They work with disabled children and adults, geriatric patients with Alzheimer's disease or perhaps Parkinson's. They are a creative and intelligent profession with lots of research behind their work and they do wonderful and amazing things!

Click here to watch a video of one of my favorite world-famous music therapists, Dr. Deforia Lane, talking about the music and breast surgery study that they conducted in Cleveland. You can also type this into your browser: https://www.surgicalserenitysolutions.com/Deforia

There are music therapists who play or sing for the patient immediately before surgery, but again, that is quite a luxury and most hospitals and clinics cannot offer this to everyone. Always ask your surgeon at the pre-op visit whether music for the patient will be provided or whether you are allowed to bring your own cordless headphones and preferred music.

The reason we created our therapeutic Surgical Serenity Solutions playlists, is so that hospitals can either stream the music directly to the patient's own headphones or Bluetooth earbuds, or they can purchase the patient-model headphones and give it to each patient to continue their recovery at home. We do offer bulk pricing to hospitals whether they purchase headphones or subscribe to our mobile app playlist.

If you choose to use music during your surgery, there is a very good chance that you will be less anxious, more relaxed and have less need for as much medication as someone who is tense and frightened about their procedure.

Depending on the type of the procedure you had, your recovery could be anywhere from a few days to several months. However long you spend recuperating, listening to our playlists or your favorite soothing, comforting music will help keep you relaxed and let your body heal faster.

When we are tense, anxious, in pain, or stressed out, our bodies are not able to mend themselves as quickly. Our bodies are intended to do most of their healing naturally. Actual physicians and nurses didn't exist thousands of years ago and yet obviously, humans have continued to survive and improve in their abilities. It is truly "survival of the fittest!"

There have always been healers, however, people who knew intuitively what to do with various symptoms and conditions. And we know from ancient legends, drawing on cave walls, and eventually, ancient treatises, that music was usually a part of healing ceremonies. Early humans used vocal toning and chanting in their healing rituals. Illness was thought to be caused by the presence of evil spirits and driving those spirits out with drums, rattles, and voices was one of the methods they used.

Today, we may be more "civilized," but music and rhythm, and conscious intention still help humans to survive and thrive in many and varied situations.

CASE HISTORY 11: Shoulder Replacement Surgery

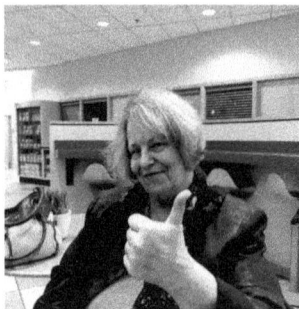

This patient had previously undergone surgery for her other shoulder to be replaced and suffered a lot of pain and discomfort with those surgeries. She wanted to do something different and had heard out the power of music through headphones.

This time, she reported that getting the headphones several weeks before her surgery and listening to the music every day, greatly relieved the pre-surgical anxiety that she always suffered. Furthermore, she was able to wear them during her shoulder surgery and avoid a general anesthesia.

During the procedure she said that the surgeons and nurses were impressed that she could answer their questions while still listening to the calming music.

When the surgery was over, she continued listening to the soothing music during the day and at night for sleeping. She also listened after her post-op physical therapy sessions when the pain had again been stirred up.

To hear her tell her story click here or type into a browser: www.surgicalserenitysolutions.com/jane

CASE HISTORY 12: Patient with Music Background Fearful of Cataract Surgery

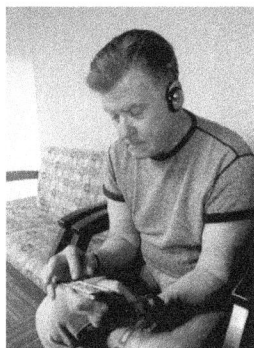

"Joe" was a 62 year-old healthy male going in for cataract surgery. He was anxious because he was in a profession where eyesight and vision are extremely important. If anything at all went awry, it could end his profession.

Another "complication," when it came to music and surgery, was that Joe had a previous life as a classical pianist and was quite familiar with classical piano repertoire and fairly critical of performances. Being a classical pianist actually is a drawback because familiarly with these pieces brings up associations that may or may not be positive.

This is why I've chosen to include unfamiliar pieces in the Surgical Serenity Solutions playlists in hopes of eliminating previous associations. During surgery, you want to just drift off to the beautiful, steady music and not think about whether you've played this piece, heard it before, or even taught the piece before.

The waiting room was packed with anxious patients, chattering away and nervously speculating on what their surgeries would be like for them on the morning of his surgery. Joe found the constant noise annoying. However, he reported that as soon as he put the headphones on and began listening to the music, he was able to focus on other things and filter out all the anxious twittering that was going on around him.

The first photo is of Joe wearing the Surgical Serenity Solutions headphones calmly listening to a playlist in the waiting room prior to surgery.

In most ambulatory care centers, patients are taken back and put in a large room with only curtains between them. It's often impossible for patients not to hear other conversations happening around them. Joe continued to wear the headphones once he was brought back and prepped into a similar environment and prepped for surgery. The headphones effectively blocked out the other conversations, yet he remained aware enough to hear when medical staff addressed him directly.

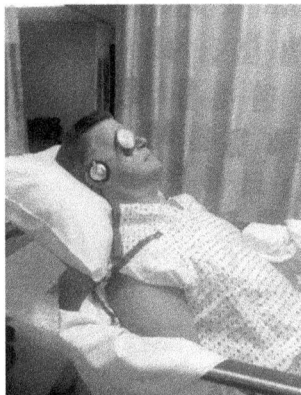

I happened to be there with Joe that day and heard a nurse say he would not be allowed to wear the headphones into surgery. I quickly explained that these cordless, pre-programmed headphones had been CREATED for surgery and were providing anxiety and pain-relieving music so that patients needed less medication. She asked the anesthesiologist to weigh in on this. He said immediately that he had read much of the recent research on benefits of music during surgery and thought it would be a great idea for Joe to wear them into surgery.

When the procedure was over, Joe slept peacefully for another 15-20 minutes. He awoke knowing exactly where he was and feeling ready to go home. (This cataract procedure took place in an ambulatory surgery center.)

Joe reported the music had been "wonderful" during the procedure and had helped him get through it with less fear of pain. He went on to say that as he was coming out of the anesthesia, it was very orienting for him to begin hearing the music again and know immediately where he was and what had just happened.

When it was all over, Joe wanted to continue listening to the music. He believed it created a "cocoon of serenity and calm" for him. He wore the headphones while I drove him home. The once-skeptical patient said he couldn't believe what a difference listening to the specially selected music through the headphones had made to the entire experience.

CHAPTER 7

What Surgeons, Anesthesiologists, and Music Therapists Say About the Benefits of Music in Surgery

So far, I've told you what patients have experienced about the process of using music with surgery. In this chapter, I share some comments by surgeons, anesthesiologists and music therapists. Their comments are specifically about Surgical Serenity Solutions headphones and music.

Sandra Elam, MD at Lifespring Inc.:

"Dr Alice Cash's earphones designed for surgery are the highest and best thing you can do for yourself if you are facing surgery. I had had a failed bowel resection (colectomy) , then an ileostomy. I was in no way prepared for those surgeries and they were terrible. Using Dr. Cash's headphones for the third and reversal surgery was a completely different experience. The surgeon as well as the anesthesiologists were impressed and said that it made their work easier!! I don't know why everybody doesn't wear them into surgery!"

Les Garson, MD, Anesthesiologist at University of CA, Irvine Medical Center (2014):

"Dr. Cash has created a valuable new addition to the surgical suite. Now patients and surgeons can benefit from music with surgery to facilitate faster, safer procedures. Bravo."

Thomas Mayo, MD, Anesthesiologist in Boston, MA:

"As an anesthesiologist with an extensive background in classical music, I am a strong proponent of Dr. Cash's headphones. Rarely, if ever, in medicine is there an intervention that has repeatedly

demonstrated efficacy in multiple studies that also carries with it virtually no risk to the patient. As a physician, I am always weighing the risks and benefits of each treatment to determine if it's worth utilizing. Surgical Serenity Headphones are unique in that they carry immense benefits without any downside. I am always pleased to accommodate a patient's wishes to bring music into the operating room. I would be particularly enthusiastic if they had these pre-programmed cordless headphones that would maximize the physiologic benefits through rhythmic entrainment. I recommend talking to your surgeon as soon as possible in the process, and certainly mention your desire to bring headphones in on the day of surgery to the anesthesia team. This would best be accomplished if you have a pre-op appointment with someone from anesthesia, but not everyone will have this chance. This could also happen during a pre-op phone call. Whenever it happens, try to be prepared to assuage any concerns or skepticism with the fact that these headphones, and music in general, have been and are currently being used in operating rooms across the planet, including many world-renowned medical centers."

Lisa Gallagher, MT-BC [board certified music therapist], Head of Music Therapy, Cleveland Clinic:

"These headphones are an ingenious solution to the delivery of music during the perioperative period. Get them for your next surgery, dental visit, or medical procedure and feel the difference!" Cleveland Clinic Head of Music Therapy, 2014

Michael Peck, MD, Anesthesiologist at Johns Hopkins Suburban Hospital:

"These surgical serenity headphones are a gift to the medical world because there are so many different places in medicine and dentistry where they can calm and soothe the patient naturally."

Scott Sugar, MD, Anesthesiologist:

"I had been thinking for a long time about how music and surgery/anesthesia could work together to help calm patients without as much anesthesia. Surgical Serenity Solutions has solved this process and has affordable, effective headphones and music waiting for the patient."

Arthur Harvey, DMA, Music for Health Services:

"I've watched the progress of this wonderful business, from idea to manifestation! Dr. Cash has created a process and a tool that will alleviate of lot of anxiety, pain, and suffering, all through the power of music! Bravo!"

David Friedman, MD, Cleveland Clinic, Florida:

"We were among the first of the 20 Cleveland Clinics to use the Surgical Serenity Solutions headphones and were so pleased that we invited Dr Cash down to our Florida hospital so that she could deliver a Grand Rounds lecture to our surgeons and anesthesiologists on her research and her patented solutions. We intend to use her mobile app, too, when it is available with our own or patient's Bluetooth headphones."

PART II

INSIGHT INTO THE HISTORY AND SCIENCE OF USING MUSIC DURING TO MEDICAL PROCEDURES

CHAPTER 8

Ancient and Contemporary Use of Music for Surgery

Medical historians tell us that the earliest evidence of surgery is from 3000 BC. Although we don't know what, if any, kinds of anesthesia might have been used, we do know that physicians in ancient Greece, Rome, Egypt, and Sumeria were well-aware of the healing powers of music and of music's ability to soothe and comfort. Physicians often prescribed live music played by local music healers for the sick patient. They recommended a specific instrument such as the lyre or the early flute be played in a specific mode, such as Dorian mode or Aeolian mode, or a certain type of voice such as soprano, alto or tenor, singing a song of a certain quality and tempo.

This was typically part of a treatment or healing procedure, so no one thought it was strange or "unscientific." The great physicians of the time knew the power that music, melody, rhythm, and timbre had and utilized it fully for what it could accomplish.

Music has been a source of healing and comfort from earliest times, and today, anthropologists, musicologists and ethnomusicologists maintain that the very earliest music, long before the Bible existed, was the music of nature. The blissful sounds of waves lapping the shore, wind in the trees, babbling brooks, and birdsongs were the earliest music. When humans began to create their own music, they were likely attempting to imitate they sounds of nature, both with their voices, but also with early instruments, such as flutes, stringed instruments and drums.

Current Use of Music with Surgery

Over the next 2000-3000 years, music as a treatment for physical and emotional ills has evolved into the current fields of music therapy, music medicine, music healing, sound healing, and even music thanatology. Music thanatology studies the benefits of music to the patient who is in the process of dying.

Music therapy and music medicine are practiced around the world, but the idea of music with surgery is still relatively new. Today, probably the majority of surgeons play music of their choice for themselves, without considering what might be best for the patient. Only in the last 25 years+ have people been looking at having music that is best for the patient.

In the 20th century, Dr. Evan O'Neil Kane first introduced a gramophone into the operating room. Medscape reports that the practice of incorporating music into clinical care soon caught on, and eventually surgeons began playing records with their own mental state in mind.

A well-known surgeon in Louisville, Kentucky told me that in 1953, he paid a woman to sit in the corner of the operating room and play 78-rpm records while he performed lengthy spine surgeries. He laughed when he said that "one patient began coming out of anesthesia prematurely while the record playing was 'When the Saints Go Marching In' and the lady was a little confused about exactly where she was at that moment. We quickly clapped the ether mask over her mouth!"

In modern times, surgeons have been playing music in the operating room since the 1940s and 1950s, but the music was usually intended for surgeons and reflected their taste in music. The generally-held belief was that the patient would be under general anesthesia and would not hear the surgeon's music or the sounds of surgery and conversations of doctors and nurses. Subsequently, hundreds of patients have come out of surgery reporting that they not only heard the surgeon's music (which they didn't like) but that they heard conversations among the medical staff which were very upsetting. One surgeon in Louisville, KY was reportedly playing the song "Another One Bites the Dust" by Queen and thought this was quite funny.

So originally, this was one of the compelling reasons that I created the headphones; so that patients could have their own best music, and the surgeon could have HIS own best music. The more that I read about all the calming and opioid-sparing benefits of slow, rhythmic music, the more I realized that this had never been done and that I could do it myself.

I realized that many patients actually DID hear upsetting conversations during their procedures and often suffered from "free-floating anxiety" as a direct result. They also heard the surgeon's chosen music which they did not necessarily like or appreciate. I decided that it would just not be that difficult to provide headphones with the patient's best type of music, in a few different genres. As time goes on, we will continue to produce more and more rhythmic entrainment playlists in genres from around the globe. (A Calypso playlist in the works now!)

CHAPTER 9
Rhythmic Entrainment Explained

I've mentioned the words "rhythmic entrainment" several times, but not many people really know what it means. Rhythmic entrainment is a very well-documented scientific phenomenon that was discovered in 1665 by a Dutch physicist named Christian Huygens. Although Huygens original experiment was with metronomes, the principles that he discovered also have applications to the human body undergoing surgery. What the concept states is that vibrating bodies in close proximity tend to synchronize and beat/pulsate in unison. Here is the definition found in Wikipedia:

> **Entrainment** in the bio-musicological sense refers to the synchronization (e.g. foot tapping) of organisms to an external perceived **rhythm** such as human music and dance. Humans are the only species for which all individuals experience **entrainment**, although there are documented examples of **entrained** nonhuman individuals.

There are different kinds of entrainment, such as the entrainment of moods or feelings, but what we're talking about is rhythmic entrainment. This occurs, when a steady rhythm or pulse, is present near a human body, in this case the patient. As a direct result of the slow, steady pulse of the music, the patient's heartbeat and rhythm begin to calm down and then synchronize with the music.

It was further discovered that even when patients are sleeping, in a coma, or under general anesthesia, the body still responds to the pulse of a nearby, steady beat. For that reason, if the patient undergoing a surgical or dental) procedure rhythmic entrainment can be obtained with slow, steady, soothing music delivered to the brain, through (preferably) cordless headphones. With headphones, the music goes directly to the brain through the eighth cranial nerve and the patient's heartrate and breathing begin to slow down and stabilize. This is the power of rhythmic entrainment.

One of the many tasks of the anesthesiologist is to monitor the vital signs of the patient to make sure the heart rate, breathing, blood pressure, and body temperature are stable. If any of these vital signs can be stabilized simply by the patient listening to music that engages rhythmic entrainment, then that is the way to go.

Entrainment in general

Rhythmic entrainment is a type of entrainment, but entrainment happens in many different settings in life. There is social entrainment, for example; when you go to a football game or other sporting event, there are cheerleaders there to whip the crowd into a frenzy of enthusiasm for their team. Getting everyone to cheer together, to sing together, to chant together. This is entrainment and here, it's the *mood* that is being entrained. Same with a rock concert, where a current pop music idol like Lady Gaga or Taylor Swift is performing. The crowd is entraining with the electric mood of the event.

Another very different example would be a church or religious service. After singing a congregational hymn or response, the attendees are feeling joined together and of a like mind. This is entrainment. When a chorus, a choir, an orchestra or a chamber ensemble experiences exact unity when performing a music work together, this is entrainment.

Not only do they entrain with each other, but they also entrain with the audience. This is one of the ways that you can tell if the performance went well. At the conclusion, the audience leaps to their feet and the performers are beaming with joy.

But until recently, the power of musical entrainment in a hospital or surgical setting has never really been explored or applied to the individual patient having surgery or other medical/dental procedures. Now when I speak to conferences and gatherings of medical personnel, they invariably say, "What a great idea! I'm surprised no one thought of this sooner!"

When a physician or nurse enters a patient examining room, one of the first things they do is to listen to the heartbeat and the lungs. Heartbeat and breathing are both involuntary processes that should be slow and rhythmic in a healthy patient. When either of these is erratic, too shallow, or too fast, the patient is NOT in a state of good health but is in a state of dis-ease. Understanding body rhythms and their reflection of health is part of the physician's job. Music can help with this.

CHAPTER 10
Music and Neurochemistry

Music affects the body, mind, and spirit in so many ways. We've talked about entrainment and rhythmic entrainment. Another way that music affects the body is through the release of neurochemicals, such as dopamine and serotonin, produced in the brain and released into the bloodstream. Both neurotransmitters help people to calm down and focus better. These are the so-called "feel-good" chemicals that many people try to produce naturally through listening to music, running, spending time with good friends and dancing, among others. These activities produce the so-called "natural high."

Then there's adrenaline, produced in the adrenal glands and released into the bloodstream and increases energy. You may ask, "You mean music can produce adrenaline?" Absolutely! Think of the two-note section of "Jaws" that always mean that the sharks are nearby and circling! It makes you want to move away quickly! Music can produce adrenaline but it's usually because there's a previous association with that music.

The neurotransmitters, serotonin and dopamine, are totally natural and utilizing them before surgery is a great idea. Listening to slow, soothing, rhythmic music in the hour or 90 minutes before surgery is a way to give yourself some of your own neurochemical relief and perhaps engage a process that is similar to the "relaxation response" and increase relaxation and calm with your own neurochemicals. This is ideal.

Oxytocin, which is produced in the brain, is released by the pituitary gland. Oxytocin is a powerful "feel-good" chemical and is typically produced when two people in love gaze at each other, when a mother looks at her infant, and when people listen to music that they love and associate with someone they love or something they love. If you can put together a list of songs you love, ones that make you think of a time when you were in love, then you can create your own playlist of songs that bring back a time in your life when you were feeling happy and in love. When you're feeling anxiety (as in the days and weeks before surgery), on the day of your surgery you can put these songs on your headphones as soon as you get to the hospital, then just close your eyes and let the waves of oxytocin melt away your anxiety.

CHAPTER 11

The Issue with Opioids

We are in an opioid crisis. Pain is an inevitable part of surgery and opioids are an effective way to treat pain. But some doctors and some patients tend to over-do it. The patient who is experiencing pain may very well say to himself, "If one is good, two are better; I can always get more!"

The doctor is thinking, "This patient is in pain and there's no need for that. I'll go ahead and provide a refill although the recommended refill isn't until after 30 days."

What neither one takes into consideration is that IF there is a genetic predisposition to addiction, this is a very easy way to unwittingly lead the patient to become dependent. This can lead to opioid addiction.

So, if the pain medication can be supplemented, or augmented, by music, you can utilize your body's serotonin, dopamine or oxytocin, engage rhythmic entrainment, and relax and stabilize the body.

Using music as an adjunct to pain medication with patients who have a history of chemical dependency is vitally important.

The problem of addiction to alcohol and drugs has been around for as long as we know. In our time, one of the few things that has helped has been the 12-step programs, which are based on accepting a belief in a Higher Power. This concept is very flexible and does not require belief in any particular God, but just "coming to believe" that somewhere in the Universe is a power greater than the addicted individual. All of that to say, that people who choose to be in recovery, voluntarily choose not to consume alcohol, or take drugs for recreational purposes.

So how does a person in recovery cope with the pain that is involved in surgery of any kind? This is a very tricky and delicate issue and it is wise to talk with both your surgeon, anesthesiologist, and your 12-step sponsor if you are the person in recovery. Obviously, music through headphones can be part of the solution. The drugs that are often administered before surgery, to calm anxiety are benzodiazepines and include things like Valium and Xanax. Both drugs are often abused. Of course, there are non-opioid anesthesia and pain medications. But if you have a history of abuse of drugs or alcohol, using a playlist specifically created to calm surgical anxiety can be an especially important part of your approach to surgery.

You'll see in many of my case histories that the patient was listening to soothing music through headphones and did not need any pre-surgical anxiety medication. Of course, you might need pain medication during and after the surgery, but even then, music through headphones has been shown to reduce pain perception by as much as 20%. See this research study: https://www.surgicalserenitysolutions.com/wp-content/uploads/2016/07/Our-SSS-study.pdf

CHAPTER 12

The Relaxation Response

In the 1970's, Dr. Herbert Benson, a professor at Harvard University, discovered a process that happens to people who are meditating. He had been studying the Transcendental Meditation technique and found that the bodies and minds of practitioners achieved a calm and peaceful state of homeostasis, wherein there is a slow, steady heartbeat, a slow, steady breathing, and a calm mind. A similar state can be achieved through music and through the process of rhythmic entrainment. The end effect of a calm mind and vital signs is much the same thing.

Listening to this music through headphones helps to achieve this state faster because it is coming directly into the brain through the eighth cranial nerve, rather than music through speakers in the room.

In an article from Stanford University [https://www.surgicalserenitysolutions.com/Stanford] it is noted:

> Recent interest in sleep, meditation and hypnosis research has spurred scientists to take a closer look at music. A small but growing body of scientific evidence suggests that music and other rhythmic stimuli can alter mental states in predictable ways and even heal damaged brains.

This article continues, "Music with a strong beat stimulates the brain and ultimately causes brainwaves to resonate in time with the rhythm, research has shown. Slow beats encourage the slow brainwaves that are associated with hypnotic or meditative states."

An article from the University of Nevada reports:
[https://www.surgicalserenitysolutions.com/Nevada]

> "A slower tempo can quiet your mind and relax your muscles, making you feel soothed while releasing the stress of the day. Music is effective for relaxation and stress management."

When patients are induced into "the relaxation response" through rhythmic entrainment, their body rhythms are moved toward homeostasis. Homeostasis is exhibited in the body in many different areas. One important area would be body temperature. When healthy, the normal body temperature is 98.6°. When ill, the body has the ability to raise that temperature, or to lower it. When healthy, the human blood pressure is around 120/80 for a female and 125/90 for a male. Music with a slow, steady beat between 50-70 per minute can assist in bringing and blood pressure that is elevated or too low into homeostasis.

Then there are parameters such as palm perspiration (which occurs with anxiety), muscle tension, and the number of inhalations and exhalations per minute. When patients are in a state of homeostasis, these bio-parameters are stable and within normal range. The proper slow, steady, and soothing music, through the process of *rhythmic entrainment,* can induce the relaxation response and then homeostasis.

Here are the four major ways that music positively affects the body during surgery:

- Rhythmic entrainment

- Relaxation

- Homeostasis

- Neurochemicals serotonin and dopamine

Now that we have taken a look at the many reasons to use music with your surgical (or medical/dental procedure) I hope you are beginning to see the logic of and necessity for an idea like pre-loaded headphones for surgery or our scientifically compiled playlists. Both the music on the pre-loaded headphones and the music on the five downloadable playlists, tap into the power of rhythmic entrainment and allow the patient's heart rate and breathing to synchronize with the music tempo. Stabilizing the patient's vital signs can be done totally with music, assuming that the patient doesn't have a pre-existing heart condition.

The playlists have been used with so many different kinds of surgery, including dental surgery and childbirth, so chances are it will work for you, too!

PART III

OF INTEREST TO HOSPITALS, CLINICS, AND MEDICAL PROFESSIONALS

CHAPTER 13

Overview for a Complete Hospital Therapeutic Music Program

Recently, I gave a presentation to the Baptist Health Hospital in Louisville, Kentucky about the benefits of a complete hospital therapeutic music program. This chapter outlines are some of the points I made.

Music in a healthcare setting is well-researched and its benefits for patients and staff is well-known. The benefits for patients, especially in the perioperative area, include:

- Reduced anxiety

- Reduced pain perception

- Reduced opioid requirements

- Reduced nausea and vomiting in recovery

- Faster discharge from recovery area and hospital

Public-Facing Benefits

Of course, the first consideration is for the patients. I call these public-facing benefits. These are:

- Patient Satisfaction scores would increase because of personal care touch and holistic treatment with latest technology

- Baptist Health Hospital would become the first hospital in Kentucky to offer therapeutic music hospital-wide through Bluetooth connection

- Baptist patients would require fewer opioids for pain through the use of music, which is a natural and effective anxiolytic agent and pain management tool

Baptist Hospital uses evidence-based practice and thousands of scientific studies recommend the use of music to reduce anxiety and the need for pain medications.

Nursing and medical staff benefits

The benefits for nursing and medical staff are equally important. These include:

- Less one-on-one time required pre-surgery (or pre-procedure) because the patient is engaged with music through headphones or earbuds

- Less time required administering medication before the procedure because the patient is calmed and soothed by the music and the rhythmic entertainment it induces

Areas of Hospital that can benefit directly from therapeutic music

Many surgical suites and procedure rooms can also benefit from therapeutic music, such as:

- Colonoscopy/Endoscopy Suites
- Labor and Delivery
- MRI
- Kidney Dialysis and Lithotripsy
- Wound care
- Chemotherapy
- NICU
- Newborn nursery
- Outpatient lab/blood draws, etc.
- Agitated ER patients
- Geriatric Use
- Behavioral health ECT

How the music is delivered

The music needs to be delivered in a way that maintains sterility, avoids cords that could interfere with the medical procedure, and obscures most sounds while allowing conscious patients to still hear statements and questions from medical personnel. For this reason, we recommend self-contained or Bluetooth headphones – or possibly earbuds.

Each room that provides patient care could have a Bluetooth-enabled device with music streamed to Bluetooth headphones or earbuds. The hospital can provide these devices for patients who want them (as the orthopedic surgery department is already doing) or patients can buy them at a pre-surgical visit.

The devices can be re-used with disposable earpiece covers.

Does this Therapeutic Music Delivery System Take the Place of
a Music Therapist?

My belief is that a therapeutic music delivery system can greatly enhance and broaden access to music therapy in a cost-effective way.

A one-on-one session with a music therapist who has created a relationship with that patient is always first choice. However, every day, hospitals around the world provide surgical and other medical procedures to patients, all of whom could benefit from the use of therapeutic music.

Providing a music therapist for each patient is not practical. However, with our carefully chosen playlists, patients can benefit independently by choosing to listen to therapeutic music delivered by personal use devices. Hospitals can easily, legally, and affordably purchase the headphones or license the music to have on hand to lend to patients. Patients will appreciate the opportunity to choose from five different music genres to maximize the benefits of rhythmic entrainment. Today, through Bluetooth technology, this is a cost-effective way for every patient to benefit from the powerful effects of therapeutic music.

Furthermore, my hope is that hospital and medical facility administrators and staff will recognize the benefits therapeutic music for patients, and that if units are not provided in-house for patient use, that patients be encouraged and supported in using their own Bluetooth device to privately access our special line of playlist apps.

It's important to note that in the recent past hospitals were using methods to deliver what they believed to be therapeutic music utilizing methods that as of January 2019, are no longer legal. This includes Apple Family Sharing, Pandora individual subscriptions, and Spotify individual subscriptions. Today hospitals must license all music for in-facility use from ASCAP, BMI, or Digital Streaming Platform (DSP), or other licensing platform.

The Surgical Serenity Solutions products are available from our website. The following playlists are featured:

- Classical Blend
- Jazz
- New Age
- Lullabies
- Memory Care

Users can select one or multiple playlists. Playlists are designed for continuous play throughout the procedure, regardless of length.

We recommend that patients listen to playlists using earbuds or headphones so that extraneous noise and conversations are eliminated.

Visit the Surgical Serenity Solutions website for direct links to purchase headphones or the app of your choice.

Click here or type this URL into your device browser: www.surgicalserenitysolutions.com/digital-products/

Purchasing from Surgical Serenity Solutions includes proper licensing for use in hospitals, ambulatory care centers, and other facilities.

Hospitals, medical facilities, and medical professionals are invited to contact Dr. Alice Cash and her team directly to discuss bulk purchases and specialty licensing Cloud Kit units. DrAlice@SurgicalSerenitySolutions.com

CHAPTER 14

Music Licensing Protocols for Hospital

Music licensing protocols for hospitals and dental facilities are largely unknown … to the hospital side of the equation. Music licensing has been around for a long time, but sadly, music is one of those things that most people believe should be free. Never mind that composers and performers spend hours and hours studying their craft and spend years and years trying to bring their music to the public.

The primary music licensing organizations are ASCAP, BMI, and SESAC. For the first time, they now have a division that is dedicated to licensing music in healthcare facilities. Many hospitals and clinics don't realize that you can't just purchase an individual subscription to Pandora, Spotify, or Apple Music, and then use that with patients in a hospital, even if you have an Apple "Family Plan".

I've previously spoken at length to the official hospital music licensing person at ASCAP in Nashville, Tennessee. She acknowledged that this is all relatively new (as of 2019), but licensing bodies are getting the word out now to hospitals that they must have licenses to play music for patients, even if patients are not being charged in any way.

Ever since the Music Modernization Act was enacted in the United States, procedures for music licensing have changed for the better. Finally, composers and performers can be paid for the hard work that they have done to produce their music that we all love and that can be healing, pain-relieving, and simply distracting (in a good way) for a patient in the hospital.

Hospitals have patients who are seriously ill and in Intensive Care. They also have patients who are basically healthy but need a knee or hip replaced. Then there are the people who are in simply for a diagnostic test, such as a colonoscopy or endoscopy. All of these patients could benefit from soothing, calming, therapeutic music. However, when people use commercial music that has not been curated and sequenced by a music medicine practitioner or music therapy professional, you're taking a chance of not getting the results you want.

And, if you're listening to music on an unlicensed version of Pandora, Spotify, or Apple Music Family Sharing, you're probably going to be listening to ads interrupting your serenity.

That's why we have created our five therapeutic playlists in a format that is licensable by hospitals and healthcare facilities. For more information, please fill out a contact form on our website.www.surgicalserenitysolutions.com/contact-us.

CHAPTER 15

Options for Delivering the Ideal Music: Headphones, Earbuds, or AirPods

For many decades now music therapists, music medicine practitioners, and even anesthesiologists, have experimented with different ways to deliver the ideal music to patients undergoing surgery. Most proved to be somewhat successful, but were either very expensive, unwieldy, or difficult to implement in various ways.

Some did not consider that the music the patient needed and the music that the surgeon wanted were usually of opposite tempo and mood. The surgeons frequently want upbeat music, music with lyrics, or music with high energy. The surgeon is attempting to keep his energy level up as well as his ability to have a laser focus. This is not at all what the patient needs. The patient is first trying to calm down his racing heart, shallow breathing, and anxious mood. The patient is looking to slow down and stabilize heart and breathing, while maintaining healthy blood pressure and body temperature.

Whether the patient is using general anesthesia, regional anesthesia, local anesthesia or no anesthesia, having a cordless method of music delivery is very important. Otherwise, cords can tangle with other equipment or pose a hinderance if the airway becomes blocked and an emergency tracheotomy is needed.

Therefore, the ideal delivery method has the following characteristics:

- It avoids cords.

- It can be used in a sterile environment.

- It obscures music used for the benefit of the medical staff.

- If the patient will be conscious, it allows the patient to hear the medical staff when necessary

If headphones are not suitable, earbuds can be used.

CASE HISTORY 13: Patient Knee Replacement Surgery Experience Using Hospital-Supplied SSS Headphones

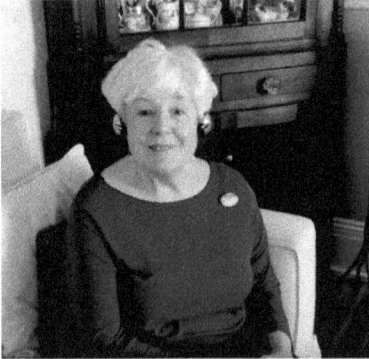

Recently, I spoke with a patient who used our new mobile app in surgery. The hospital provided Bluetooth headphones, which they now use for all joint replacement procedures, and she said it worked perfectly.

"Dr Cash, I just wanted to tell you that the Surgical Serenity Solutions worked beautifully, and the anesthesiologist and nurses came back after the operation (knee replacement) to ask about your sound program. I am so grateful to you and your wonderful creation! It did everything as promised … peace of mind!"

P.S. I think it's great that hospitals now have Bluetooth headphones waiting for the patient having surgery!

– Alice Covell, Louisville, KY.

Listen to Alice Covell tell her story in her own words.

Click here or type into a browser:
https://www.surgicalserenitysolutions.com/AliceKnee

CHAPTER 16

Current Research on the Benefits
of Music in Surgery

One of the most exciting aspects of music and surgery is that there is so much research to back up the concept. Research on the benefits of music with surgery comes from many disciplines. The fields of surgery, anesthesiology, nursing, social work, and music therapy all have wonderful research journals with studies on surgery with music.

Music before, during and after surgery or any medical/dental procedure is an excellent idea and one that should be implemented in every hospital and clinic around the world. Ideally, patients are given a choice of the genre of music they want to use, and then, within that genre, they will be given the music that has the slow, steady tempo of the healthy, resting heartbeat and that is physically calming and emotionally calming.

On August 17, 2015, the *Journal of Clinical Oncology* published the findings of a research study trial titled, "Effects of Music Therapy on Anesthesia Requirements and Anxiety in Women Undergoing Ambulatory Breast Surgery for Cancer Diagnosis and Treatment: A Randomized Controlled Trial.

Click here to access the online article or type this into a browser: www.surgicalserenitysolutions.com/defo

The trial was headed up by music therapist Deforia Lane, PhD, MT-BC. She begins the Introduction by acknowledging:

> Women who are undergoing surgery for breast cancer diagnosis and treatment often experience heightened

anxiety. Although surgical anxiety may be managed by administering larger dosages of anxiolytic drugs, these drugs can depress circulation and respiration, making nondrug alternatives particularly attractive.

Dr. Lane concludes that adding music therapy to the perioperative period could greatly improve the surgical experience and give the patient a sense of control when everything else might seem so out of control. Their study used both 5 minutes of live music, chosen by the patient and performed at bedside by the music therapist, or recorded music chosen by the therapists during the procedure. This study did not use music in the recovery area.

Another thing that this study demonstrates is that having preloaded headphones of your own is a more likely way to ensure that YOU can benefit for the soothing effects of music. The likelihood that any hospital in the country will have a music therapist for each patient having a procedure is extremely slim.

In 2015, Surgical Serenity Solutions had a study done on its headphones and proprietary music published in an international journal of anesthesia. In the published study, available at https://www.surgicalserenitysolutions.com/wp-content/uploads/2016/07/Our-SSS-study.pdf.

The study was conducted at and with the cooperation of the Robley Rex VA Hospital in Louisville, Kentucky. The population was men between 18-75 who were undergoing major abdominal surgery. I could not be one of the researchers (since objectivity would be compromised) and concerned that these military veterans might not be that fond of classical music. As a matter of fact, I was told that they would prefer classic rock.

The problem with that is two-fold. One, classic rock music has lyrics and most of the research indicates that purely instrumental music is best for complete relaxation and for inducing rhythmic entrainment. The second issue is that music from the mid-to-late 20th century is not in the public domain so must be purchased and licensed by the hospital. The hospital did not want to do that, nor allocate the required funds which could have been substantial.

The anesthesiologist who conducted the study said that when obtaining consent from each subject, some of whom had music in their headphones, and some who didn't, she explained to each man that the music on the headphones was the best music to engage rhythmic entrainment and, of course, she explained what this meant.

At the conclusion of the study, the most prominent and exciting finding was that pain perception decreased by 20 percent among participants. This is a very significant amount of pain reduction, and especially in a time when the opioid crisis is raging and medical professionals are searching desperately for non-addictive pain management.

Even now, several years later, people are dying in frighteningly high numbers because of addiction to heroin, fentanyl, and other opioid drugs. The Opioid Crisis could possibly be partially stopped or at least slowed down by using music for pain management and anxiety management. Music through headphones is even more powerful because it creates a "sonic cocoon" that shuts out the world temporarily, and replaces it with beautiful, soothing, steady music.

Table 1 explains how the subjects rated their pain:

| Time Point | Average Pain Score (VAS) | |
	With Music	Without Music
Arrival in recovery room	2.37	4.15
After 30 minutes	3.04	5.48
After 23 hours	2.15	4.37

[Table 1] VAS means they measured their pain with a Visual Analog Scale

Table 2 shows how much pain they felt when they arrived in the recovery room, after 30 minutes, and after 23 hours. Very interesting, don't you think? Clearly, music can make a huge difference!

| Time Point | Opioids administered (morphine equivalents) | |
	With Music	Without Music
Arrival in recovery room	36.56	37.2
After 30 minutes	4.57	4.85
After 23 hours	25.18	30.36

[Table 2] Patients with music required less opioids

After this study was completed, the hospital purchased 100 pre-loaded headphones. Hospitals around the world are now using them, and some are testing the new Surgical Serenity Solutions mobile app. [https://www.surgicalserenitysolutions.com/buyanapp]

In August of 2015, a wonderful <u>meta-analysis of over 4000 other</u> studies on music and surgery was published in the British Journal, The Lancet. This was a huge endeavor. The study can be accessed here:

<u>www.SurgicalSerenitySolutions.com/Lancet</u>

The publication begins with a summary:

> Music is a non-invasive, safe, and inexpensive intervention that can be delivered easily and successfully. We did a systematic review and meta-analysis to assess whether music improves recovery after surgical procedures.

This meta-analysis was focusing on Phase 3 of the perioperative period, the recovery room phase.

The Endearing Words of Martin Luther King

Many of us would agree with Martin Luther King's when he said, "My heart … has often been solaced and refreshed by music when sick and weary."

If that solace can happen in our private lives, why not in hospitals? Companies have profited from the mood-altering effects of music, but medicine has been much slower to reap the benefits. Hopefully, the accumulating evidence base might change that.

Unfortunately, due skepticism or disinterest driven, perhaps, by results of some studies that show only incremental positive change, change to embrace the therapeutic benefits of music are slow in coming. But music is a simple and cheap intervention, which reduces transient discomforts for many patients undergoing surgery. A drug with similar effects might generate substantial marketing and use. How sad.

The world has benefitted for millennia from the mood-altering power of music. The greater public arena has paid millions of dollars to hear specific performers and ensembles live and paid millions more for their recordings. Yet the field of medicine has been exceedingly slow to recognize the therapeutic benefits of music. Starting in the area of surgery, I am passionately trying to change that!

Here is a link to a <u>dozen plus clinical research studies</u> that were done on music with surgery over the last 25 years around the world. Invariably, the researchers determined that music can significantly decrease anxiety levels in the patient, decrease pain perception throughout the perioperative period, and decrease nausea and vomiting in recovery, as well as aid in orientation to time and place after surgery.

[www.surgicalserenitysolutions.com/medical-research]

CHAPTER 17

Next Steps

I hope that this book has helped you and taken away some of the fear and anxiety that you had!! Remember that music is one of the most ancient ways of calming and soothing the mind and body.

Here are some steps you can take:

- Download our questionnaire to use during your pre-surgical visit:
https://www.surgicalserenitysolutions.com/free-checklist

- Purchase your own headphones with your preferred genre of specially chosen music here:
www.surgicalserenitysolutions.com/digital-products/

- Purchase our app for your smartphone. Get more information here:
https://www.surgicalserenitysolutions.com/buyanapp

- Watch our video testimonials here: (yes, misspelling is correct for link)
https://www.surgicalserenitysolutions.com/video-testimonals

- Read additional written testimonials here:
https://www.surgicalserenitysolutions.com/written-testimonials

Keep the music playing!

ACKNOWLEDGMENTS

I'd like to thank the following individuals for their valuable wisdom, insight, help, and support:

Dr Crystal Sahner for pointing out to me, in 1995, that there was little or no information for the general public about Music with Surgery. As a music therapist and health psychologist she convinced me that I needed to provide this information to the millions of people having surgery and other medical/dental procedures.

Dr Michael B Hudnall for reading and formatting/editing many versions of this manuscript.

Ms. Nonie Hudnall for posing for many pictures, when wearing the headphones for her multiple surgeries. Also, for her encouragement and support when things were moving slowly.

Mrs. Alice Adelaide Hudnall for her emotional and financial support of this project when we weren't sure it would ever get off the ground.

Ann and Stewart Cobb for their unflagging emotional and very generous financial support of everything related to Surgical Serenity Solutions. None of this would have been possible without your help.

Dr. Marina Varbanova for conducting the clinical trial on our Surgical Serenity Solutions headphones with our pre-loaded proprietary music, analyzing the data, and getting it published in a professional journal of anesthesia research.

Mr. Jonathan Goldman for donating one of his powerful New Age playlists to Surgical Serenity Solutions and being a tireless advocate for our process and the results it brings.

Dr. Ellen Britt for believing in this idea over 10 years ago and giving me opportunities to be on her webinars to talk about Surgical Serenity and answer call-in questions.

Ms. Kat Sturtz for being a patient and supportive editor of this book. Though we both suffered health challenges while editing was in progress, we used music of all kinds to heal and repeatedly get back to the job at hand. Thanks also to her for great help with marketing the book.

Ms. Ellen Finkelstein for being my online business coach and tireless encourager. I could not have done it without you!

LIST OF CASE HISTORIES

Chapter 6

CASE HISTORY 11: Shoulder Replacement Surgery

CASE HISTORY 12: Patient with Music Background Fearful of Cataract Surgery

Chapter 15

CASE HISTORY 13: Patient Knee Replacement Surgery Experience Using Hospital-Supplied SSS Headphones

MORE ABOUT DR. ALICE CASH

Dr. Alice Cash is one of the world's few clinical musicologists. Based in Louisville, Kentucky, USA, she brings to her work over 40 years of professional experience as a college professor, clinical therapist, solo and chamber music performer and composer.

Since 1990, Dr. Cash has been in the field of Music Medicine and conducted clinical research at the University of Louisville School of Medicine, under the guidance of Dr. Joel Elkes, Dr. Leah Dickstein, and Dr. Rif El-Mallakh. Her clinical work at the University of Louisville lead to her career in music medicine.

In addition to her work with the University of Louisville, Dr. Cash lead the development of using music a hospital setting at Baptist East Hospital, Louisville, KY. She has founded 3 companies: Healing Music Enterprises, Surgical Serenity Solutions and Crescent Hill Counseling.

In 2008, Dr. Cash received a United States patent on her unique process for using music in the perioperative process. Today her pre-programmed headphones are being used in leading hospitals in the U.S. and other countries.

A downloadable version of her full Curriculum Vitae is available from the About Us page on her website: www.surgicalserenitysolutions.com/about-us/

Here are some highlights:

FOUNDER:

- Healing Music Enterprises
- Surgical Serenity Music & Headphones
- Crescent Hill Counseling

EDUCATION

- M.S.S.W. -- Kent School of Social Work; University of Louisville, Clinical Focus

- Ph.D. -- Musicology

- Post-grad Musicology and Performance

- European Study in Italy, Piano Performance with Prof. Ilonka Deckers

- Masters Music -- Piano Performance, University of Louisville

TEACHING EXPERIENCE

- Healing Music Academy, Louisville, Kentucky full spectrum of online and classroom courses

- Adjunct Faculty, Kent School of Social Work, University of Louisville, Louisville, Kentucky.

- Guest lecturer in the Department of Expressive Therapies, Division of Allied Health, University of Louisville. Guest lecturer in Department of Psychiatry and Behavioral Sciences, School of Medicine, University of Louisville.

- Adjunct Professor of Piano, Indiana University Southeast, New Albany, IN

- Assistant Professor of Music, University of Kentucky, Jefferson Community College, Louisville, KY

- Instructor in Church Music, Southern Baptist Theological Seminary, Louisville, KY

- Assistant Professor of Music, Central Wesleyan College, Central, SC

SURGICAL SERENITY MUSIC AND HEADPHONES

- U.S. Patent awarded for a process of using music during surgery.

- Winner of the "Venture Sharks" competition for best new business idea and innovation. Venture Club of Louisville.

- Grand Rounds Presentation at University Hospital, Louisville, KY "Music as an Adjunct to Anesthesia"

- Grand Rounds Presentation at Cleveland Clinic Florida, "Music as an Adjunct to Anesthesia: a review of recent research" (included two solo piano recitals in hospital, before and after Grand Rounds).

- "The Power of Music during Surgery" a lecture/recital at Second Presbyterian Church, Louisville, KY.

ARTS IN MEDICINE EXPERIENCE

- Research Associate in Music/Medicine (under Dr. Joel Elkes) Genesis Center, University of Louisville School of Medicine, Department of Psychiatry, Division of Attitudinal and Behavioral Medicine, Louisville, KY Research in music/medicine with emphasis on the healing powers of tone and breath. Projects included: "Arts and the Elderly": Dr. Jane Thibault, Dr. Alice Cash, and Dr. Vija Lusebrink. "The Effects of Group Singing with Severely Disturbed Children": Dr. Adam Blatner and Dr. Alice Cash. Dr. "The Psychophysiological Benefits of Chant": Dr. Kathy Smith, Dr. Alice Cash, Dr. Anita Maiste, and Dr. Paul Salmon. Expressive Therapies Department: Education on Toning and Chanting. "Toning with chronic pain patients" at Genesis Clinic: Dr. Clifford Kuhn and Dr. Alice Cash. "The Psychophysiological Effects of Gregorian Chant": Dr. Alice Cash, Dr. Anita Maiste, and Father Columba Kelly.

Research Projects at Baptist Hospital East

Professional License

- Kentucky Licensed Clinical Social Worker

Clinical Experience

- Healing Music Enterprises and Crescent Hill Counseling, Owner and Clinical Director: oversee all therapy and provide services to individuals, couple, and groups. Administer and teach Healing Music Academy classes on subjects from "Music and the Brain," to "Music and Alzheimer's Disease."

- Baptist Hospital East, Behavioral Health Family Therapist; specializing in issues of chemical dependency, sexual addiction and sexual health and consultant in Music Medicine

- Norton Psychiatric In-patient unit: Conduct music-centered psychotherapy groups; PRN social work

- Norton Out-patient Clinic: work with individuals, couples, and families using brief solution focused therapy, music and imagery, and other expressive and traditional psychotherapies.

- Child Evaluation Center, Department of Pediatrics, School of Medicine, University of Louisville: developing a music therapy program for children with autism; including assessment and therapy.

- Coordinator of Music and Medicine; closed program for the Arts in Medicine; transferred clients and programs to other clinical locations.

- Genesis Center, Department of Psychiatry and Behavioral Science: work with dissociative, depressed, anxiety and panic disorders and families in crisis. Led weekly group for music centered psychotherapy.

- Bingham Child Guidance Clinic, University of Louisville, Department of Psychiatry and Behavioral Science: psychotherapy with children and families utilizing brief solution-focused therapy, expressive therapies and cognitive/behavioral therapy.

- Hurstbourne Care Center: provided clinical music therapy services, individual and group, as part of a study on the effects of music with Alzheimer's patients.

- Our Lady of Peace Psychiatric Hospital: music-centered psychotherapy, including toning and chanting with individuals and groups in the "impaired clergy" program, a program for clergy suffering from various mental disorders and/or substance abuse. Coordinator of Music and Medicine University of Louisville, School of Medicine, Department of Psychiatry

- Coordination of two major research projects: "The Therapeutic Use of Music with Alzheimer's Disease" and "Psychophysiological aspects of Chant." Completed Research Studies in Music Medicine

- "Psychophysiological Aspects of Chant" 1992. Conducted by Drs. Cash, Salmon, Maiste, and Elkes

- "The Effects of An Individualized Music Stimulation Program on Alzheimer's Patients" 1993. Conducted by Drs. Cash, Salmon, and Maiste

- "Music and Thought Organization" 1995. Conducted by Drs. Cash and El-Mallakh Completed Research Studies in Music Medicine

Training in Music/Medicine

- Phoenix, AZ: Intensive training workshop with Dr. Alfred Tomatis from Paris on the "Healing Powers of Gregorian Chant." Included 80 hours of lecture, assessment and training.

- Coursework through the Institute for Music, Health, and Education: Level I: Curative Aspects of Breath and Tone (54 CMTE credits) Level II: Healing Properties of Color, Tone, and Breath (32 CMTE credits) Level III: Assessment of Health through Advanced Applications of Breath, Tone, and Color. (36 CMTE credits)

- Advanced and Accelerated Research Issues in Contemporary Music Therapy: focus on the use of music in a modern hospital setting, the use of guided imagery with music, and the history of the therapeutic uses of music.(on-going)

- Institute for Music, Health and Education, Boulder, CO. Mastering Classes on above subjects with Don Campbell and Laurie Rugenstein, RMT-BC, co-directors of the institute.

- Mastering Level Intensives in Toning, Boulder, CO.

- Therapeutic Sound School with Don Campbell in Wilkes Barre, PA.

- Mastering Level Intensive in Toning, Boulder, CO.

ADDITIONALLY:

- Has presented dozens of professional workshops, lectures, and recitals, plus and published hundreds of professional papers

- Has made dozens of major media appearances and interviews, including NPR, PBS, CNBC, and NBC Nightly News

To book Dr. Alice H. Cash or other inquiries:

Dr. Alice H. Cash

2822 Frankfort Avenue

Louisville, KY 40206

DrAlice@HealingMusicEnterprises.com

Phone: 502-419-1698 FAX: 502-895-7688

The Surgical Serenity Solutions products are available from our website. The following playlists are featured:

- Classical Blend

- Jazz

- New Age

- Lullabies

- Memory Care

Users can select one or multiple playlists. Playlists are designed for continuous play throughout the procedure, regardless of length.

We recommend that patients listen to playlists using earbuds or headphones so that extraneous noise and conversations are eliminated.

Visit the Surgical Serenity Solutions website for direct links to purchase headphones or the app of your choice.

Click here or type this URL into your device browser: www.surgicalserenitysolutions.com/digital-products/

Purchasing from Surgical Serenity Solutions includes proper licensing for use in hospitals, ambulatory care centers, and other facilities.

Hospitals, medical facilities, and medical professionals are invited to contact Dr. Alice Cash and her team directly to discuss bulk purchases and specialty licensing Cloud Kit units. DrAlice@SurgicalSerenitySolutions.com

www.ingramcontent.com/pod-product-compliance
Lightning Source LLC
Chambersburg PA
CBHW022044190326
41520CB00008B/696